Holding On

....

Anthropology of Contemporary North America

Holding On

African American Women Surviving HIV/AIDS

Alyson O'Daniel

University of Nebraska Press

Lincoln and London

Portions of chapter 3 previously appeared in "Access to Medical Care Is Not the Problem: Low-Income Status and Health Care Needs among HIV-Positive African American Women in Urban North Carolina," *Human Organization* 70, no. 4 (2011): 416–26. Reprinted with permission.

Portions of chapter 6 previously appeared in "'They Read [the Truth] in Your Blood': African American Women and Perceptions of HIV Health," *Medical Anthropology: Cross-Cultural Studies in Health and Illness* 33, no. 4 (2014): 318–34. Available online at http://www.tandfonline.com /doi/abs/10.1080/01459740.2013.808636.

Library of Congress Cataloging-in-Publication Data
Names: O'Daniel, Alyson.
Title: Holding on: African American women surviving HIV/ AIDS / Alyson O'Daniel.
Other titles: African American women surviving HIV/AIDS
Description: Lincoln: University of Nebraska Press, [2016]
Series: Anthropology of contemporary North America
Includes bibliographical references and index.
Identifiers: LCCN 2015043383 (print)
LCCN 2016000124 (ebook)
ISBN 9780803269613 (pbk.: alk. paper)
ISBN 9780803288409 (epub)
ISBN 9780803288416 (mobi)
ISBN 9780803288423 (pdf)
Subjects: LCSH: AIDS (Disease)—Treatment—United States. | African American women—Medical care.
Minority women—Medical care—United States.
Minorities—Medical care—United States.
Classification: LCC RA643.83 .O33 2016 (print) | LCC RA643.83 (ebook) | DDC 362.19697/920082—dc23
LC record available at http://lccn.loc.gov/2015043383

Set in ITC Charter by Rachel Gould.

For *Charlie*, *Delia*, and *Wren*,
my heart;
and for *Lola*,
my inspiration

Contents

Tables

Acknowledgments

In some ways this book represents part of my life's journey. I am fortunate and grateful to have so many caring and supportive people lighting my path. First and foremost I would like to thank the women of Midway and the Health Partnership employees whose life experiences form the heart of this book. I am deeply thankful for your generosity, candor, and willingness to teach me about services and survival. I am also deeply thankful for the many personal kindnesses you all extended to me. Fieldwork can be lonely and frustrating at times, and many of you offered cheer and friendship when I needed them most. For all your insights, patience, and kindheartedness, thank you. It was truly a privilege working with you all.

This study would never have been possible without the guidance and encouragement of Mary Anglin, Deborah Crooks, Karen Tice, Erin Koch, and Monica Udvardy. From study design to analysis and write-up, their feedback and advice were always thoughtful and helpful, oftentimes prompting me to dig deeper, think harder, and write more clearly. Even when amid calls for rethinking and revision, each was encouraging. I cannot thank you enough for all that you've done to help me achieve this goal. Mary Anglin deserves particular and special recognition. As my mentor she challenged me at every opportunity, in the end helping me to become a more thorough and careful scholar. For all this and for modeling inspired scholarship, I thank you.

Special acknowledgments also go to the many colleagues and friends who have provided feedback and support as I was writing this book. I was lucky to have many incredible scholars willing to lend their time and expertise to reading and critiquing this manuscript. Sabrina Chase and Alisse Waterston offered feedback more helpful than I had any right to expect. Their suggestions for change greatly improved the quality of my writing and this book. Rebecca Adkins-Fletcher, Greg Reinhardt, and Krista Latham also provided crucial feedback on portions of the manuscript, often accepting the request with little time for turnaround. Series editors James Bielo and Carrie Lane, former University of Nebraska Press editor Derek Krissoff, and current University of Nebraska Press editor Alicia Christensen also offered especially useful feedback on the manuscript and the publication process. Their professionalism, patience, and encouragement were particularly helpful and appreciated as this uninitiated author navigated the various stages of book publication. Thank you, as well, to Vicki Chamlee for her wonderful copyediting and to Sara Springsteen for guiding me through the end stages of book revision. To each of these generous colleagues, I am sincerely grateful for your help on this journey. Any remaining errors are mine alone.

Rebecca Adkins Fletcher, Maureen Meyers, Cindy Isenhour, and Jenny Williams offered the kind of support only the dearest of friends can. Each offered advice concerning writing sample chapters and "shopping" the prospectus. Their advice is appreciated and indeed helped bring this book to fruition. What I am most grateful for is their friendship. Each has been at times the comedian, confidante, counselor, and cheerleader that I needed. You are amazing colleagues and even better friends. Thank you.

Anyone who knows me well understands that my family has been a monumental source of support in the research for and writing of this book. To my mom and Brad, who have always believed I would publish a book, and to my dad and Lynne, who have my second-grade short story framed, thank you for all that you've done for me and for always believing in me. I am lucky to have such supportive parents. To my sister, Jennifer, and my brothers, Jeff, Nick, and Ryan, thanks for being so fun and for not allowing me to take myself too seriously. Going home is one of my favorite trips to make because of you all and the lovely young people you're raising. To Betty and Joe, thank you for all your encouragement over the last ten years and, most important, thank you for Charlie. Charlie, Delia, and Wren have been amazing and constant sources of love and support. Charlie has been a true partner in this journey, and Delia and Wren are the brightest stars lighting our path. There truly aren't words to express how thankful I am for each of you. You are my heart.

Funds for this research were provided by the National Science Foundation (Dissertation Improvement Grant [PI Mary Anglin, Co-PI Alyson O'Daniel], BCS 0823572) and the University of Indianapolis.

Author's Note

Throughout this book I capitalize the labels "Black" and "White." I do so because, as applied here, the labels refer to social and political categories of people who are differently positioned in relation to White supremacism and historically driven processes of structural inequality. These terms are therefore not intended as mere descriptors of skin color, or what is commonly referred to as race. Capitalizing these terms is not only a reflection of social processes and experiences of identity *and* subjectivity but also a recognition of the shared history among group members within an unequal and unjust social system organized by race.

Holding On

Introduction

In 2009 I sat with Lady E. in an HIV/AIDS service organization's conference room as she described a recent relapse in her recovery from drug
addiction. Her hands shook as we talked, perhaps as a result of with-
drawal but certainly as an effect of the fear she felt concerning her health
and well-being. "I lost my apartment and missed my opportunity for
Section 8. I smoked up all of my Social Security back pay. I was smoking
day and night. I was defecating and vomiting. I had smoked so much
quality cocaine that it had stripped the membranes in my mouth. So I
couldn't eat. My throat didn't work. I went nine days with no food. I could
put the food in my mouth and chew it up, but I didn't have enough juices
to swallow it. I know all of this was because I was having a pity party."

As Lady E. recounted the details of her two-week crack binge, I began
to wonder how a woman so intimately connected to the local system of
public health care could slip through the cracks as quickly as she did. I
wondered, too, what it meant that Lady E. considered her relapse as a
personal failure. After spending more than a year in the low-income
communities of Midway, North Carolina, I knew well the strategies that
drug dealers used when looking to hold their consumers captive. Offering a "free taste" had proven particularly effective for sabotaging an
overstressed and underserved HIV-positive woman's recovery plans. I
also knew that Section 8 housing was indeed a scarce resource that
many women, whose daily life realities were incompatible with policy-
mandated eligibility procedures, lost. Still I was surprised that Lady E.
had stumbled on what she described as "the path to wellness."

Over the course of sixteen months, Lady E. had made dramatic changes to her life with the help of newly defined, federally funded HIV/AIDS care and related U.S. Department of Health and Human Services programs. In the fall of 2007 local care programs began implementing new policy pronouncements associated with the 2006 Treatment Modernization Act (TMA). Increased funding for the state of North Carolina had translated into a slate of new programmatic services and information-sharing networks aimed at meeting the "comprehensive and intensive" needs of HIV-positive individuals. Like all of the women in this study, Lady E. was quickly integrated into a burgeoning system of care. She began attending daily substance abuse support classes, was enrolled and participated in mental health services, saw an internal medicine physician regularly, utilized nonmedical case management services, and frequently drew from the myriad financial and in-kind resources available at Health Partnership, the local federally funded HIV/AIDS service organization in Midway. With the help of these new health care programs, she saw steady improvements in her health, including her HIV disease, diabetes, and symptoms of heart disease. When I last left Midway in November 2008, Lady E. was well on her way to realizing her goals of long-term sobriety, Section 8 housing, and improved quality of life. Not seven months later, she had again hit "rock bottom." All one could do, Lady E. later told me, was to "survive by holding on to the truth of your life."

Lady E. often talked about the truth of life as though it were self-evident. She once told me in a conversation about women and AIDS, "This is the truth of your life: take the medication or don't." Initially I thought the meaning of her statement was simple. Her "truth," as I understood it, ultimately lay in recognizing her potential vulnerability to HIV-related mortality. It wasn't until much later that I realized the truth also referred to a need to demonstrate personal responsibility for health in a cultural context fraught with concerns over deservedness and moral belonging. Public HIV/AIDS care use, to put it bluntly, had become enmeshed with moral values and sentiments prioritizing individualism, self-help, and self-sufficiency. I soon learned that the truth involved with deciding to "take the medicine or don't" referred to processes of blame and conditions of survival much broader than the scope of an individual woman's mortality. In that statement Lady E. had laid bare for me an unarticulated social site structuring the lives of HIV-positive African American women using federally funded HIV/AIDS care services. No longer a cultural construction "hidden in plain sight" (Di Leonardo 1998, 10; Martin 2012, 25), survival suddenly seemed open for exploration as a paradoxical and historically contingent process wherein cultural and political economic forces met.

This book is an ethnography of survival with HIV disease. At its heart reside the daily life circumstances, experiences, and perceptions of forty HIV-positive, low-income African American women who were enrolled in federally funded HIV/AIDS care at the start of my formal study activities in November 2007. In a total of eighteen months between November 2007 and May 2012, I explored women's lives and survival experiences in relation to HIV disease and health care through ethnographic techniques of participant observation and in-depth interviewing. What unfolds in the following pages is the story of both how their lives and health care outcomes were differentially structured by material conditions of poverty and inequality and how women's experiences of health and health care came to be shaped by material conditions of global neoliberalism and associated discourses and practices of deservedness and moral belonging.

Anthropologists have broadly used the term "neoliberalism" as a key concept for making sense of inequality in the contemporary world (Richland 2009). In general the term refers to a market-based ideology and model of governance that promotes economic globalization as the most logical way to address global poverty and inequality (World Health Organization 2015). Central to this ideology of governance is the belief that "wasteful" or inefficient social spending, "excessive" government regulation, and overreliance on principles of redistribution and social values associated with public good hamper economic growth (Goode and Maskovsky 2001). Market-based models of governance have therefore involved trade liberalization, labor market restructuring, and the privatization and/or retrenchment of publicly funded programs (Goode 2002a; Harvey 2005; Jing 2006; O'Manique 2004; Piven 2001). These strategies for economic development have been accompanied by an emphasis on the social values of personal responsibility, individualism, and self-regulation, all of which are based on the idea that poverty results from an individual's failure to adapt to the demands of the market. This focus on the individual discourages collective political and economic responses to the inequality that shapes poverty (Cox 1998; Morgen and Maskovsky 2003, 317).

The global spread of neoliberal governance has had far-reaching effects. In just a few decades it has consolidated corporate and elite power at the same time it has deepened poverty and inequality worldwide (Harvey 2005, 19; Goode and Maskovsky 2001, 4). It has also realigned notions of democracy and fairness with principles of economic entrepreneurship (Di Leonardo 2008), and it has reframed human rights in the language of the global marketplace (Englund 2006). Under conditions of market-based governance, states have become guarantors of economic security and well-being largely insofar as they operate to reduce government spending on social programs and roll back policies and practices believed to "interfere" with business and trade (Ferguson 2006, 106; Goode and Maskovsky 2001). In other words, the role of the state is to provide for citizens via the maintenance of free market capitalism.

In the United States generally, and for the women of Midway specifically, the devolution of state-supported antipoverty programs has posed formidable challenges to the abilities of poor and near-poor populations to achieve daily life stability. Long before I arrived at Health Partnership, the women in this study grappled with conditions of economic globalization. For example, their economic well-being was complicated in the 1990s by trade liberalization insofar as it resulted in the movement of local textile- and furniture-manufacturing jobs overseas, a reality that increased competition for other locally available low-skill work (North Carolina Rural Center 2009). The women's vulnerability to unemployment and poverty was further complicated by the "planned shrinkage" of U.S. social programs as social safety net resources grew scarce under conditions of welfare reform (Davis 2004; Goode 2002a). To put it bluntly, by the time of this research, many of the women at Health Partnership had long ago become "hard-to-reach clients" in the language of welfare case managers because they experienced persistent poverty and chronic barriers to employment (Morgen, Acker, and Weigt 2010, xii).

Yet as this analysis attests, poor and HIV-positive women were not completely without options. Public HIV/AIDS care became for many women in Midway the de facto safety net in an era of growing unemployment and declining welfare services. This was possible because while neoliberal governance may be partially characterized by the divestment of state-sponsored antipoverty programs, it has also ushered in an era of *increased* interest in public funding for HIV/AIDS prevention and care (Susser 2009). The result has been a global scale-up of HIV/AIDS care organized around the understanding that the global HIV/AIDS pandemic is a development problem that threatens international security, free market capitalism (O'Manique 2004), and, ultimately, Western imperialism (Susser 2009).

Currently the thrust of anthropological research concerning HIV/AIDS treatment is to document the role of care programs under conditions of economic globalization (Booth 2004; Kalofonos 2010; Nguyen 2010; Susser 2009). One trend has been to examine how public HIV/AIDS care transforms impoverished and HIV-positive populations into "biopolitical subjects" and/or therapeutic citizens (Biehl 2004; Nguyen 2010), meaning that there are populations of people who become visible to the state and reap material rewards of citizenship largely, if not solely, via their adherence to state-sanctioned biomedical practices and narratives of HIV health and disease. Members of these populations are sometimes known as "biological citizens" because their disease diagnoses and disease management strategies are what grant them rights to resources from a state that is otherwise organized by principles of individualism and economic entrepreneurship (Petryna 2002; Rose and Novas 2005). In resource-poor settings (especially in developing nations), anthropologists have found that health programs for HIV/AIDS represent one of the few remaining, if precarious, tethers between state resources and impoverished citizens.

Yet despite a dramatic scale-up of the American HIV/AIDS care safety net and its increasing importance for women living in poverty, little has been said about the social effects of this public health intervention and its relationship to an American model of market-based governance. What political economic contingencies shaped the scaling up and restructuring of U.S. HIV/AIDS care? How do changes to public HIV/AIDS care work in the contexts of women's daily lives? How do the changes affect women's health? What strategies do women have for navigating new terrains of public HIV/AIDS care? In the chapters that follow, I consider these questions in relation to local understandings and practices of "survival," an often-used but under-explored notion in the social sciences.

In this book I trace the interconnected pathways of women's daily lives, public health policy, and Health Partnership care programs, drawing attention to the complicated relationships between women's living conditions, their senses of survival as lived experience, their use of survival as a cultural resource, and the programmatic service requirement to track and report survival in the quantitative terms of epidemiology, biomedicine, and fiscal reform. Amid the material stresses and emotional pains of chronic poverty, drug addiction, mental health instability, and neighborhood violence, the forty HIV-positive women in this study conceived of and took steps toward conditions they imagined would constitute life as they desired it. For them survival represented personal circumstances, emotional transformation, and intentional efforts to achieve financial stability and social mobility. Care providers, in contrast, were prompted by public health policy mandates to define survival sans the details of daily life that women found important; instead, service providers focused on factors such as length of time since diagnosis, behavioral change, blood quantification reporting, and programmatic service expenditures. By unraveling these sometimes-competing discourses of survival, I illuminate the particular policy mechanisms by which women's health and daily life stability were differentially supported and, in many cases, thwarted.

Critical Medical Anthropology

This study was conceived from the premise that health is a political issue (see Cohen 1999; Doyal 1995; Kim et al. 2000; Morgen 2002; Navarro 2004; Roberts 1997). Seen in this way, the HIV/AIDS epidemic provides a lens that broadens our grasp of social change, power relations, and the workings of contemporary social inequality. This book is accordingly grounded in the tools and insights of political economic medical anthropology, meaning I contextualize women's lives in relationship to historically specific global processes of power surrounding sickness and health care (Morsy 1996, 27). Unraveling dynamics of power in this setting required that I explore political and economic processes extending beyond HIV/AIDS and African American women in this setting.

To do so I contextualize the study participants' experiences and life circumstances in relation to welfare reform, transformations to federal HIV-related public health policy, and local social practices shaping conditions of programmatic services, including how service providers may exercise power in ways mediating women's chances for health and well-being (Baer, Singer, and Susser 1997; Castro and Singer 2004). Unraveling how power operates in this public health care setting thus means that I necessarily expand my view beyond HIV/AIDS and HIV-positive women. The lens through which I tell this story magnifies how the women's experiences of survival are shaped by processes, perspectives, and values associated with global capitalist expansion. I contend that changes in federal HIV/AIDS care policy are best interpreted against broader trends of neoliberalism described previously, including the retrenchment of welfare programs, opposing class interests, and the popular belief that poverty results from individual deficits in behavior.

Black Feminist Perspectives

At the same time, this ethnographic account examines the interplay between the systems-level processes described earlier and the micro contexts of the women's daily lives. I do so by paying explicit attention to often-ignored social differences among poor African American women living with HIV disease. Although they are often assumed to represent a coherent epidemiological population, here I demonstrate that HIV-positive Black women must also be understood as socially diverse and variably positioned actors who transform, contest, and consolidate relations of privilege and subordination through their health experiences and strategies. This text thus is unabashedly indebted to tools and insights of third-wave feminist analysis that rejects the notion of universal feminine identity. Instead, I follow the insights of scholars such as Kimberlé Crenshaw, Leith Mullings, Faye Harrison, and Irma McLaurin who have positioned processes of race, class, and sexuality as central to gender identity and gendered experience. I specifically draw from intersectionality theory to consider interactive and multiplicative effects of race, class, and gender in relation to women's life circumstances (Crenshaw 1989). Proponents of intersectionality theory—for example, Brodkin (2000), Collins (1990), McClaurin (2001), Morsy (1993), and Mullings and Schulz (2005)—reject the idea that one aspect of social difference, such as gender, may alone explain sources of oppression, identity, or health disparity. They instead explore how gender, race, and class are experienced as concurrent, making clear the pathways by which they connect and affect Black women's chances for health (Weber 2006; Zambrana and Dill 2006, 196). Under this framework and in this book, race, class, and gender are consistently viewed as simultaneously oppressive social processes, combining in various health-related ways that are always historical and contextual (Bolles 2001, 34; Caldwell, Guthrie, and Jackson 2006, 164).

Contrary to traditional public health approaches to HIV/AIDS, this intersectional approach to health and disease asserts that the mutual construction of race, class, and gender makes it difficult to measure any one category's contribution to experiences of disease. Scholars exploring the intersectional nature of HIV/AIDS emphasize the political and economic complexities structuring women's access to care and chances for health and survival. Collins (2001), for example, considers the interactive and multiplicative effects of race, class, and gender in relation to new forms of racism characterizing post–civil rights era America. She explores how African American men and women are both affected by racism in health-demoting, yet gender-specific, ways. Her work spotlights how economic globalization, labor market restructuring, and associated ideologies of color blindness connect with historically driven and class-based stereotypes concerning Black sexuality, masculinity, and femininity. She argues, in turn, that these stereotypes obscure poverty's systemic roots and thereby justify racial disparities in access to the means for health.

Cohen (1999) has also written about how identity politics have shaped and stratified Black community responses to HIV/AIDS. She begins with the long-held assertion that dominant institutions manipulate gender, class, and racial identities in ways constituting the "special category" of delinquent poor women of color (see also Bridges 2011). Her work explores how popular notions of "deficient" Black Americans structure Black institutional responses to HIV/AIDS. Cohen illustrates that HIV/

AIDS-related work in Black communities involves a multiplicity of identities, definitions of membership, locations of power, and strategies for the political, social, and economic survival of the community. Thus HIV/AIDS, as an issue disproportionately affecting only certain segments of the African American population, shapes experiences of racial identity as well as identities constructed around gender, sexuality, and class. For this reason, argues Cohen, it has historically not been embraced as part of what she terms "the Black political agenda."

Berger (2004) further examines this notion of intra-community difference and employs the concept "intersectional stigma" to focus attention on how HIV seropositivity is experienced in light of already stigmatized racial, class, and gendered identities. She asserts that "stigma" is largely an informal mechanism of social exclusion, whereas "marginality" is a structural concept. "Stigma" thus denotes more than institutionally based discrimination or disadvantage; indeed, it is fundamentally about how people relate to one another and justify exclusion. From this vantage point, Berger argues that HIV-positive Black women, prior to their positive diagnoses, occupied disadvantageous social locations that rendered them as already vulnerable to exclusion. HIV disease compounds their identities, culminating in a qualitatively distinct set of experiences. Thus seropositivity constitutes another interlocking axis of identity-shaping experiences of ill health and disease.

Taken together these analyses replace one-dimensional portraits of Black women as community-minded and invisible caregivers (see Schiller 1993), pragmatic strategists (Battle 1997; Williams 2003), organization builders (Stoller 1998), and "institutional allies" or strategists on behalf of others. Instead, these works portray how the realities of Black women's lives are varied and contingent. They also assert that there can be no single category "women" or even "Black women" who are uniformly oppressed by the same conditions and who thus share the same health experiences and health care outcomes (Mohanty 1991). In my estimation these analyses remind health researchers to consider how categories of race, class, and gender differentially structure distributions of disease within and between populations, as well as how they shape institutional definitions of and responses to population health. *Holding On* takes seriously the charge to dispel the idea that historically given definitions of female "Blackness" offer an appropriate way to delimit a public health population and address their health care needs. Instead, this analysis considers in fine detail the uneven effects of health care policy and programmatic services protocol across gradients of poverty and social differences that I observed among Black women surviving with HIV disease.

Study Methods

The methodological approach used in this study is based on a commonly shared conviction among anthropologists: while I may have expertise in cultural and medical anthropology, only the women with whom I worked are experts on their experiences of survival. This belief led me to consider, in a variety of ways, how to centrally position the women's perspectives in the research design and any subsequent analyses. I sought to build research relationships based on a foundation of trust and mutual respect. Despite my good intentions, however, the tasks of study recruitment and retention were onerous and, at times, downright stressful. As members of an under-studied and over-stereotyped group who were acutely aware of their socially marginal place in society, many of the women with whom I sought to work were sensitive to the idea that my career would, in some ways, be built on their backs, so to speak. For example, on a September morning in 2007, I sat in the lobby of Health Partnership, waiting to talk with the director of client services. My goal that morning was to explain my research project to one of Midway's HIV/AIDS community gatekeepers and, hopefully, secure her permission to work with her agency. I came to the director that morning by way of a local, university-affiliated public policy researcher who had been kind enough to introduce us via email just a few days before. I had been in Midway for two months at this point and had failed to generate the contacts I needed for this work. It seemed that everyone I had met during previous preparatory visits to Midway no longer worked in the community. As I nervously waited in the lobby, the receptionist made small talk by asking if I were a prospective volunteer or a pharmaceutical sales representative. Presumably my outsider status, my Whiteness, and my business casual clothing led her to assume that I was not a potential client. When I explained to her that I was a researcher planning to conduct a study in the community, a woman I would later come to know as Raquel exclaimed, "Aw, hell nah! I'm not talking to any researcher!" She promptly left the room while audibly muttering about White people as she left. I sat bewildered and embarrassed by Raquel's public and unequivocal rejection.

That morning I did meet my goal of securing Health Partnership's formal support for this project, yet I knew the challenges of realizing this research plan were only beginning. Raquel's blatant disinterest in my presence signaled to me that I would have to work very hard to recruit and build rapport with study participants who would be willing to talk candidly with me about their lives. For this reason participant observation at Health Partnership became the focus of my earliest research activities. Once I obtained permission from my university's Institutional Review Board to begin the study, I conducted participant observation at the organization four to five days a week. At first my activities were confined to the agency's lobby, and I then gradually extended them to internal spaces such as conference rooms and client and staff lounges. Staff frequently asked me to help with small tasks such as stapling handouts and unloading equipment and food shipments from delivery trucks. I gladly lent a hand wherever I had permission to be and, slowly, began asking questions about the agency and its services. Before long, employees seemed to better understand my interest in working *with* Health Partnership as means of gaining insight into the local provision of federally administered health resources. They were generous and patient with me as I prompted them to provide me with what amounted to a crash course on agency history, HIV/AIDS health care policy, and programmatic services provision.

My activities as a participant-observer at Health Partnership were also designed to facilitate meeting HIV-positive women. I thus also worked *through* Health Partnership, using it as a kind of research "home" where I could recruit study participants. Through the organization the women eventually came to know me as a researcher, as a volunteer, and, in many cases, as a person with life circumstances and responsibilities outside of the project. The organization's waiting area and client lounge hosted most of my first acquaintances with research participants and our many subsequent conversations. Many of the women with whom I worked were not employed or were only sporadically employed. Health Partnership, in these contexts, was a regular stopover for women searching for ways to combat boredom, anxiety, addiction cravings, or loneliness. Most staff members maintained an informal atmosphere that translated into a community space where the organization's clients could stop in unannounced for companionship, advice, and entertainment. I spent many afternoons sitting in the parking lot of the organization, smoking cigarettes, laughing, and talking with the women in this study.

In some cases the women I had come to know well asked to drive around town while we chatted about their lives; my having a car was definitely an asset in this setting. I learned on these drives about some of the unapparent public places the women frequented, the various neighborhoods in which they had lived, and the challenges they faced for meeting their basic needs. In three cases these afternoon drives culminated in some women giving me a tour of the various locations around town where they had encountered physical violence. It was through these excursions that I really began to learn how the women made sense of their neighborhoods and the city.

A few months into the project, I began conducting regular and intensive participant observation with six women. This development meant our meetings had moved from Health Partnership into their homes and other daily life spaces. This group of women ended up reflecting the diversity of the interview sample with respect to their socioeconomic circumstances and their length of time since diagnosis. We spent countless hours running errands, window shopping, observing and discussing neighborhood dynamics, and generally just hanging out in their homes. I also less regularly conducted participant observation outside of Health Partnership with an additional eleven women. These opportunities usually arose in response to special programs and sporadic invitations to attend an agency-affiliated support group. Such instances provided an invaluable means of getting to know those women who only occasionally frequented Health Partnership. Special events and support group meetings also allowed for a more nuanced assessment of the varying ways in which the women received the messages and advice of health care professionals and event sponsors.

My commitment to participant observation as a methodology in this setting eventually facilitated the kind of in-depth interviewing I had hoped it would. As is characteristic of many studies among difficult-to-reach populations, I recruited interview participants through firsthand meetings at Health Partnership and through word of mouth. I asked study participants who I felt trusted me to lend "word of mouth" to this project. Their willingness to promote the project to others helped me establish trust with participants who were otherwise skeptical of my presence in the community. This type of "snowball sampling" also allowed me to better grasp the varying social circles and networks among women enrolled in Health Partnership programs.

During the initial 2007–8 fieldwork year, I conducted a first round of interviews with forty HIV-positive African American women, all of whom were older than eighteen years of age. Interviews broadly assessed the women's socioeconomic circumstances, including their histories of incarceration, addiction, and mental illness. I closely followed an interview guide, and each interview lasted, on average, an hour and fifteen minutes. About halfway through the initial fieldwork period, I began second interviews with women from the primary interview group. Because I was better established in the community by this time and had been able to form closer working relationships with many of the women in this study, my secondary interviews were more collaborative than the primary interviews were. By collaborative, I mean that the women seemed to feel more open to refining my questions and taking the interviews into directions that they felt were appropriate given their life contexts. This dynamic improved on the original interview guide, particularly given that the secondary interviews were concerned with the women's perceptions of HIV disease and disease management. Twenty-seven women participated in this part of the project.

A third set of interviews during this initial fieldwork year concentrated on better understanding the experiences of Health Partnership employees. I completed interviews with ten care providers and the organization's executive director. These interviews explored the dynamics of care from the perspectives of care providers, including their experiences with policy changes and services transformation under conditions associated with the 2006 TMA.

While experiences lived and recounted during the 2007–8 research year provide the foundation for this ethnography, my interpretations of the women's lives and my understanding of the significance of HIV/AIDS policy change were elaborated and refined during two subsequent follow-up research periods. From May to June 2009, I conducted follow-up interviews with ten women from the primary interview group. I selected interview respondents based on insufficiencies I felt needed elaboration in the original field record I created from field notes and interview transcripts. I also chose follow-up interview respondents who had potentially life-altering events unfolding at the time I exited the field in 2008. Questions focused on recording changes in the women's living conditions, health needs, and strategies for achieving stability. During this time I continued participant observation in the women's daily life spaces and at Health Partnership. These opportunities allowed me to assess changes in the women's living conditions. I was also able to document modifications in support service provision protocol, as the new fiscal year had ushered in further policy amendments and agency transformation.

I returned to Midway for a final month of research in May 2012. This trip proved logistically difficult because many women with whom I had previously worked had been "lost to care," meaning they no longer accessed health services funded by the Ryan White Comprehensive AIDS Resources Emergency Act. And given the instability of their lives, the phone numbers and addresses I had updated in 2009 were no longer accurate. I reconnected with the few women I could find but spent most of the time I had discussing agency changes with the four remaining Health Partnership employees who had participated in the initial research and were still employed as HIV/AIDS care providers in Midway. While employees could only speculate why specific study participants stopped seeking help from Health Partnership, their assessments of services and policy change brought to light increasingly restrictive policies and procedures that may have discouraged the women from seeking further help.

Ethnography and Daily Life

Overall the methods I employed for this study did lend themselves to in-depth exploration of women's daily lives. The narrative I present is heavily shaped by the personal perspectives and opinions of the study participants. That is, the analysis I have constructed reflects material conditions, social circumstances, and life moments that the women perceived as important to their experiences of survival with HIV disease. In this way the events examined here amplify the women's voices and perspectives in the way that I had hoped. Yet I also draw from my own position within this community and from my perceptions and analyses as a cultural and medical anthropologist particularly attuned to issues of social inequality. For this reason the story I tell here is equally one shaped by the micro-political contexts of fieldwork as I understood them through the analytical lenses of my discipline.

As Abu-Lughod reminds us in *Veiled Sentiments* (1986), "who we are" while in the field matters. The information and experiences to which I was privy reflected the participants' understandings of our social similarities and differences. In ways sometimes funny and sometimes disconcerting, my identity as a young, White, female researcher circumscribed this work. I wish that I could discuss how I became an honorary "insider" in Midway's HIV-positive community. I secretly hoped that I would somehow manage to elide the boundaries of race and class to find a space outside of power where there would be true sharing between the researcher and the researched. I knew this was not really possible. Yet while in the field I often thought about how I could communicate my feelings of solidarity with those women with whom I worked. I did know, however, that such a display could produce resentment, discomfort, and quite possibly laughter. While I tried very hard to appreciate and understand what women were telling me, I knew that my own privilege shot through every question I asked, every prompt I offered, and every interpretation I made. I became conscious of the "White metaphor" I might be reinforcing as a White researcher conducting this particular study with Black participants.

In some contexts I was the researcher asking questions, listening intently, making clarifications, and taking notes. This role was always circumscribed by my race, my age, my economic background, and my gender. Women would sometimes assume that I was unfamiliar with historical circumstances such as welfare reform because of my age and my presumed economic background. Women sometimes also assumed that I would be uncomfortable and vulnerable in their homes and neighborhoods. As one research participant stated in a phone call to confirm our later interview appointment, "You're like a moving target in the 'hood. Call me when you get here, and I'll walk you from your car." Truth be told, sometimes I did feel out of place in the women's homes and vulnerable in their neighborhoods. As I performed and sometimes fumbled through my role as a researcher, the women were gracious and patient community hosts—even if they had an occasional laugh at my expense.

In informal contexts I was a young White woman who had not yet learned how to respond to the women's banter. For example, two research participants called me "Similac" (a commercial brand of infant formula) until, months later, I responded by calling them "Metamucil" and "Bengay." With much laughter and a hug, Metamucil responded that Midway was "toughening" me. More than once Bengay joked that I would return home "poppin' and lockin' and better for it." These short dialogues were pivotal in this set of relationships, but they did not redefine who I was in the field. Indeed, throughout the study, some women seemed eager to put me in my place as an outsider by calling me such names as "White girl," "skinny ass," and "little momma." The name-calling, I still believe, was not meant to hurt my feelings. It performed a much more important function: it served as a reminder that the privilege of studying the women's lives was contingent upon their good will, patience, and willingness to engage with anthropological research methods.

Throughout the course of this research, many women recognized that my privileged identity could be useful to them in a service professional context. Women often asked me to speak on their behalf to social service professionals. Thus at times I performed the role of intermediary in the public health care system. Privilege operated in this milieu in strange ways. Social service professionals accepted without question when I vouched for appointments so that women could get free bus tickets. I also confirmed household crises so women could get extra food from the food pantry without question. In this capacity I helped women reschedule their missed appointments and was even asked to ensure one woman's timely admission to one of the local hospitals. I was always eager to help in this way, but I often fretted over what my role as a "voucher" potentially said about the racial and class dynamics at play. In some cases I believe service providers felt that my research relationships with clients validated the women's claims. I was, after all, "in the know" because I spent time with the women in their homes and neighborhoods. My status as a university-trained professional also lent credibility to the support I offered the women. In other cases it is possible that service providers felt self-conscious about seeming uncompassionate or inflexible to a researcher. Perhaps sometimes care providers understood my research activities as surveillance. These various roles that I assumed in the field enhanced my ability to witness and understand the women's daily lives.

Over the course of this research, eliciting health and survival experiences through the lenses of these varied positions helped to me to see the importance of study participants' life trajectories in relation to health and health care outcomes. Lady E.'s recovery relapse, for example, was not an isolated event. It was, instead, one outcome of a series of interwoven processes bearing down on a woman overburdened by conditions of poverty and inequality. Her relapse, as this book attests, is most intelligible when read against the backdrop of typically ignored details concerning the daily life conditions under which she navigated the terrains of sobriety and disease management. It is through the subtle social, economic, medical, and material details of her life that one may fully comprehend her plight. It is also through these details that one may appreciate her creativity, ingenuity, and resilience. Thus here I examine fine details of social differences among HIV-positive, low-income Black women in order to make visible the often-unaddressed complexities of health and survival with HIV disease.

Toward Unpacking Survival

Anthropological research concerning experiences of HIV survival in the United States has been slow; however, there is a long tradition of survival-centered work from anthropologists working in and with marginalized communities more generally. This scholarship reflects the commonly held notion that there is more to survival than "just" continuing to live (Hill 1991). Yet as with studies of violence until the mid-1990s, research addressing the notion of survival has been undertaken without asking the question of what survival *is*. Until now little attention has been given to varied definitions and notions of survival, how these definitions and notions may work in context, and, in some cases, how they may hide some dimensions of life while making others hyper visible. Survival, in other words, may be as unfixed, flexible, and transformative as the people who materialize it (see Robben and Nordstrom 1995, 4–6; Scheper-Hughes and Bourgois 2003).

Much anthropology concerning survival emphasizes life realities as experienced in marginal communities. For example, the publication of Stack's (1974) ethnography of an urban Black community was a timely assertion that survival, perhaps above all else, attests to expressions of agency amid constraint. Stack's ethnography clarifies how kin-based strategies of poor, urban Black families in a Chicago neighborhood increased their access to resources in a discursive and material environment that was insensitive to the needs and pragmatic concerns of impoverished populations. Her work appreciates such efforts as swapping material goods, child keeping, and recognizing mutual obligation as adaptive strategies. That is, Stack defines "strategies for survival" as actions that facilitate the satisfaction of basic needs. Survival itself, in turn, comes to be defined through the process of high-effort coping, which sustains life. In other words, to survive is to create and utilize alternative or unsanctioned means for satisfying basic human needs in contexts of material want.

This particular dimension or understanding of survival has been well used and elaborated in relation to America's HIV/AIDS epidemic. An unspoken but powerful anthropological elaboration of survival as a dimension of health took off in the early 1990s with the social-scientific emphasis on discerning the social contexts of viral transmission and infection among the poor. For example, researchers such as Pivnick et al. (1994), Singer (1991), Sobo (1999), Sterk (1999), and Waterston (1997) illuminate how, under conditions of chronic and severe material deprivation, illicit drug use and sex-for-drugs exchanges provide a means for income generation, emotional escape, and social network expansion. In the case of survival sex, survival highlights how sexual decision making may hinge on life-and-death circumstances and/or economic distress (Wojcicki 2002). Thus as strategies for survival, drug use and sex work may operate to mitigate some conditions of poverty even while paradoxically increasing the parties' vulnerability to HIV infection. Survival in this sense encompasses Stack's (1974) analysis of high-effort coping but reframes the act of coping in relation to unintended consequences such as disease transmission risk. Survival, then, also encompasses a prioritization of needs based on their perceived immediacy to risk of peril and/or death (Connors 1996).

Anthropologists such as Mullings (2005) and Chase (2011) further illustrate that survival and survivorship entail resilience, which involves not just the struggle to live under oppressive conditions but also the ability to transform conditions of constraint into conditions of possibility. It is a simultaneous recognition of the constraints posed by "historically created relationships of differential distribution of resources, privilege and power, of advantage and disadvantage" (Mullings 2005b, 79), as well as the activism, strategizing, and everyday acts of resistance characterizing the lives of individuals and groups suffering the effects of inequality. As Hill (1991, 126) explains, stories of survival "attest to human cruelty, but equally to human perseverance." Thus our attention shifts from the facts of continuing to live and strategies for prolonging life to complex and meaning-centered processes of social existence. As the experiences and perceptions of the women with whom I worked make clear, to survive is first to perceive a struggle and then to act in and on the social world that denies the realities of that struggle. A robust theory of survival then requires building an intellectual reality that attends to the notion in all its political, social, psychological, and material complexities. We thus must begin to unpack the question of what survival is and does in order to understand what survival means.

I begin here with the basic assertion that the anthropological literature on survival, though dormant it may be, makes clear that the concept is meaningful in ethnographically specific ways and thus must be understood in terms more complicated than its binary relationship to death. What does it mean to survive in contexts of HIV disease? Under what material and ideological conditions do HIV-positive women relate to the notion? What agenda does survival, as discourse and experience, serve? What can women's experiences tell us about the realities, political machinations, and processes of power at play in HIV-related survival? *Holding On* examines these questions by tracing the social and material structures circumscribing women's lives, experiences, and perceptions of HIV-related health.

Organization of the Book

I offer this book as one concrete step toward understanding how survival is currently used in HIV-related health policy circles as well as how women struggling with health policy changes and daily life experience it. This book is an argument for an in-depth ethnographic examination of an often-used but under-examined concept in relation to inequality and public health policy. It constitutes survival as both a field site and a paradox that require exploration in relation to profound shifts in the contemporary U.S. political economy of health and health care. My intention here is to ignite in the social sciences a serious discussion of survival as a theoretical concept *and* as a social process and system of meaning intractably tethered to processes of power, inequality, and transformation. Thus I do not offer a theory of survival but instead a discursive opening from which to examine the possibility of seeing how survival operates in realms of health care, support services, and daily life. As this account demonstrates, experiences of survival among poor Black women living with HIV disease have much to teach us about how cultural transformation engenders novel forms of success and failure in public health policy and programs.

I begin this inquiry in chapter 1 by tracing transformations in AIDS-related health and human service programs and in federal legislation specific to the use of and eligibility for HIV/AIDS care services so as to present a long-term view of the political and material contexts structuring the lives of Black women living with HIV disease. I specifically examine the conditions under which poor and near-poor populations have experienced the erosion of state-funded social safety net programs while at the same time there has been substantial investment in and commitment to funding for HIV/AIDS prevention and care. Central to this undertaking is examining the epidemiological course of HIV/AIDS in the United States, as well as popular discourses circumscribing the epidemic and the populations widely understood to be at increased risk for infection. I highlight the emergence of relationships between popular and racialized discourses of deservedness, welfare reform measures, and federally mandated restrictions in how HIV/AIDS care dollars may be distributed and spent at the local level.

In chapter 2 I present an overview of the institutional and community contexts of the lives of the women in my study. I describe the structure and content of Midway's system of HIV/AIDS care, paying particular attention to how national public health care policy changes were implemented in Midway's local system of care. Using interviews and participant observation with Health Partnership employees, I take pertinent verbatim statements from these records and examine how ambiguities of policy pronouncements led service providers to utilize informal and exclusionary criteria regarding eligibility for services. Interwoven throughout this description is an analysis of the ways in which employees' personal life circumstances and educational training shaped their strategies for relating to and either serving or denying the needs HIV-positive women.

Chapters 3, 4, 5, and 6 are ethnographic accounts centered on my field research among HIV-positive women enrolled in Health Partnership programs. In chapter 3 I examine social and material differences among Black women living with HIV disease in order to more broadly consider variability vis-à-vis housing status and quality, strategies for income generation, substance abuse and mental health issues, histories of incarceration, and the viability of their personal social networks. Drawn from the women's experiences at home, with their families, in their neighborhoods, among friends, and in the public spaces they frequent, this chapter examines in depth the gradations of poverty and their significance for determining health care needs and priorities.

Chapter 4 takes up the public health–related educational contexts of the women's lives, highlighting how and where they learned about and experienced biomedical and epidemiological definitions and notions of survival. Using ethnographic examples of techniques and processes of moral instruction as well as the women's engagement with lessons of morality and social worth, I assess how the women were taught to regard survival with HIV disease as a medical event divorced from the material and social disadvantages in their lives at the same time that they were paradoxically saddled with the responsibility to become economically self-sufficient.

Chapter 5, in turn, examines the women's differential engagement with the lessons on survival in relation to the differences among them that are highlighted in chapter 3. Through an ethnographic examination of how the women's abilities to perform, or exhibit, the necessary behavioral change and to personalize support service networks mattered for their access to support and the satisfaction of daily life needs, I consider the ways in which the women's differences were defined and made to matter in the context of HIV/AIDS care programming. I take up the notion of "social network surrogacy" to amplify the impact of these variances on the women's experiences with care and to focus more finely on the women's distinct abilities to draw on policy-driven notions of survival in health-promoting ways.

The sixth and final ethnographic chapter continues to explore the women's performances of survival discourse, spotlighting how they both conformed to and resisted narrowly conceived medical understandings of HIV health and survival. Drawing primarily from in-depth interviews concerning perceptions of health and daily life with the virus, this chapter examines alternative discourses and bodily schematics through which the women asserted context-specific conceptualizations of health and survival. When read against the backdrop of policy change and social network surrogacy, the women's understandings of the relationships between life circumstances and health invite novel means of tracking HIV health care outcomes and the empowerment of women living with the virus.

The conclusion pulls together this sequence of health care contexts as part of a critical anthropology of survival. An important part of this ethnography questions how to merge the political, social, psychological, and material complexities of survival unraveled here with the practical concerns of providing public health and programmatic services. I argue that narrowly defined biomedical definitions of health, health care, and survival must be balanced with policies amenable to helping variably situated women reach their goals of social transformation and upward mobility.

1. "Other" Stories of Social Policy and HIV Survival

> If you go back to the history of what [the Ryan White CARE Act] was
> even based on, go back to the name—"Comprehensive AIDS Resources
> Emergency Act." It was for an emergency. It wasn't planned on being a
> thirty-year infrastructure-building project. It was designed to be a "oh
> crap, we got a crisis. What do we do for these people that are dying
> and are all going to die?" So start with that as your premise, and you
> can see how we've come to this problem.
>
> JEREMY, Health Partnership executive director

In the summer of 2012 I met with Jeremy, the recently appointed executive director of Health Partnership. I had come to visit Jeremy on this
day largely as a formality. I had returned to Midway, North Carolina, in
hopes of reconnecting with several women with whom I'd previously
worked. I had already spoken with a few service providers from the
agency and felt I understood the latest changes to organizational policy
and services provision. Still I thought it appropriate to reconnect with
agency administrative officers, especially given that my last conversations with Jeremy were prior to his appointment as executive director.

Jeremy had long been involved with the organization as the director
of development. Many times I had observed his leadership skills at high-
dollar fund-raisers held to solicit donations from local middle- and upper-
class allies of the HIV/AIDS community. I'd also occasionally witnessed
his humorous performances as an emcee for the agency's monthly Drag
Queen Bingo fund-raiser. I knew through my observations at these and
other events that he was a remarkable and passionate advocate for people living with HIV/AIDS. I also knew he had an impressive grasp of the
policy changes and advocacy initiatives characterizing the state's pub-

lic health response to the epidemic, for our few informal conversations in years past had centered on local advocacy initiatives related to HIV/AIDS. What I had yet to discuss with him, however, was his personal experience with HIV survival as an HIV-positive gay man who came of age in the late 1980s and as an active participant in the national political processes circumscribing federal care programming. Throughout our talk that day, he heatedly recalled political battles concerning HIV/AIDS programs, taking care to pay his respects to contemporary HIV/AIDS legislative policy architects and allies such as Ted Kennedy, Hillary Clinton, and Alabama senator Richard Burr. Citing several instances where continued support for federal programmatic services was in question, Jeremy framed nationwide systems of care as a "built environment" that he had personally helped to design and implement. He specifically iterated, however, that the whole idea of federally funded HIV/AIDS care had been "developed on the back of thousands and thousands of people who have died—those who didn't survive long enough to see our government do right." Vividly portraying his sense of personal investment and the "noise" he had helped make concerning a historical lack of HIV/AIDS resources in the South, Jeremy emphasized his emotional and intellectual connections to Health Partnership. As a lobbyist, as a service organization employee, as a consumer of HIV/AIDS care, and as a *human being* (his emphasis), Jeremy was committed to "speaking for those who are afraid to speak or even *survive* this disease because of the stigma." I was especially surprised when, near the end of our discussion, he disclosed that he was leaving the agency in search of another advocacy opportunity. The political contests circumscribing federally funded care, it seemed, had become as of late too difficult for this advocate to navigate from inside Health Partnership.

HIV/AIDS care has long been a political battlefield, in part because of its articulation with controversies, rules, and "universes of discourse" associated with broader American political and economic inequalities (Treichler 1999, 10). HIV/AIDS care, in other words, is not *just* about treatment and prevention of a biological disease state; it also represents a site through which the American people, institutions, and legislators enact beliefs and practices concerning social responsibility and "which kinds of lives society will support" (Geertz 2000, 93). Put simply HIV/ AIDS care is a socially constructed practice that, when analyzed in relation to broader social trends and discourses, can tell us about the workings of power in contemporary America. Illuminating processes of power in this context, however, requires us to look beyond what we think we know about it. As Treichler (1999, 15) explains, "Our social constructions of AIDS . . . are not based on objective, scientifically determined 'reality' but on what we are told about this reality."

This chapter examines changes in federal HIV/AIDS care legislation at specific moments along the trajectory of the epidemic. I connect changes in HIV/AIDS programming to conditions associated with the U.S. transition to a market-based model of governance, bringing into view the ideologies, policies, and practices broadly shaping women's experiences of HIV/AIDS care and survival with HIV disease. I therefore suspend the federal government's characterization of the U.S. HIV/AIDS treatment apparatus as a "modern public health miracle" with a "legacy of care" to consider what remains hidden when understandings of HIV-related programmatic services are narrowed to the fiscal and enumerative terms so often the focus of public discussion concerning medically indigent populations (Health Resources and Services Administration [HRSA] 2010, 3). Recognizing that the Ryan White Comprehensive AIDS Resources Emergency (CARE) Act is indeed a costly and, in many ways, highly effective public health intervention, I nevertheless consider ways in which the act has come to be entangled with questions of social belonging and historically given dynamics of racism and gender inequality. Within this exploration, I pay particular attention to how welfare reform and discourses of deservedness have subtly shaped HIV-related connotations and use of "survival," a public health concept seldom interrogated as "socially productive" in the sense that it has engendered particular forms of sociality (Comaroff 2007, 203). Survival becomes clearer as a contextually specific social construction when examined in relation to U.S. welfare reform and racialized discourses of productivity and citizenship fueling popular support of efforts to retrench antipoverty programmatic services. Such a perspective spotlights that while federal HIV/AIDS care programs may be lauded for providing crucial supports for some of the most vulnerable members of American society, they may be also critically evaluated for their role in reproducing pre-existing racial and gender inequities and health care inequality.

The Early Years: Ryan White CARE Act Legislation

U.S. HIV/AIDS care programs have been largely omitted from conversations concerning the effects of global neoliberalism (for exceptions, see Farmer, Connors, and Simmons 1996 and Susser 2009).[1] They have also been largely excluded from analyses of U.S. Department of Health and Human Services (USDHHS) policy reform (O'Daniel 2009). This is perhaps because U.S. HIV/AIDS care programs are increasingly well funded by the Ryan White CARE Act, whereas the general trend has been toward disinvestment from other social services. However, close examination of HIV-related programming and policy makes clear that federal HIV/AIDS care has indeed been aligned, in many ways, with market-friendly values and practices.

The Ryan White CARE Act is a federal funding mechanism specifically designed for comprehensive management of the epidemic among impoverished and medically underserved populations in the United States. It was enacted in 1990 to address the health care needs of people infected with the human immunodeficiency virus. The act represents the culmination of relentless activist struggle and sustained community mobilization over the course of a decade wrought with fear, grief, anger, and perseverance (Aggleton, Davies, and Hart 1997; Epstein 1996; Speretta and McAlpin 2014). Gaining federal support for HIV/AIDS care programming was a hard-won victory that the George H. W. Bush administration initially opposed because of its focus on a single disease and the precedent that disease-specific support might set for other public health populations (HRSA 2014a). Opposition also came from many other politicians and countless Americans who had denied and/or learned about HIV/AIDS via little media coverage and, in later years, inaccurate and sensational media reporting (Epstein 1996; Shilts 1987; Treichler 1999). To put it bluntly, for many, federal support for HIV/AIDS care constituted an unwelcome investment in socially marginalized and stigmatized populations (Cohen 1999; Treichler 1999).

In the early 1980s the association of HIV/AIDS with marginalized subpopulations of people paved the way for the construction of misleading (and moralizing) public health HIV/AIDS "risk groups": hemophiliacs, homosexuals, heroin users, and Haitians (Treichler 1999). The association of HIV/AIDS with specific populations of people, rather than in terms of conditions of risk, articulated with predominant social sensibilities and popular morality in troubling ways. The "risk group mentality" and the static social identities it presupposed had the disastrous effect of obscuring HIV infection in women, children, and heterosexual men (Farmer, Connors, and Simmons 1996; Ward 1993). It also misled the public about structural conditions of HIV infection and divorced public conversations concerning the epidemic from its sociopolitical and economic context (Rodriguez 1997; Act Up/NY Women and AIDS Book Group 1990; Susser 2009). This had the effect of rendering growing infection rates among women of color as invisible while isolating HIV-positive gay men as *the* problem with which the American public had to contend (Goldstein 1997). Homophobia, racism, and elitism, combined with denial and a general lack of knowledge concerning HIV transmission, led many health experts, mainstream news outlets, and the general American public to project their worst fears onto those living with HIV disease. HIV/AIDS quickly became known as a disease of the "other"; it was a disease belonging to "a community of pariahs" (Sontag 1990, 113). Thus HIV/AIDS was feared for its inevitably fatal medical prognosis as well as the social marginality that its diagnosis implied. People who shared needles and/or engaged in anal sex and unprotected sex—activities viewed as inherent to their presumably nonnormative lifestyle (Sontag 1990, 113)—were popularly believed to have "paid a fatal price" for their indiscretions (cited in Farmer 1996, 4). Risk of infection and the disease itself became synonymous with stigmatized behaviors of individuals and groups long considered as "the wretched of the earth" (Barnett and Whiteside 2002, 7). HIV-positive individuals were thus seen as blameworthy, or at fault for their disease and a rapidly accelerating epidemic.

In this context grassroots activists such as the Act Up/NY Women and AIDS Book Group and the Women and AIDS Resource Network began campaigns of self-empowerment, consciousness-raising, and self-advocacy. Self-identified "People with AIDS" claimed their right to be treated with dignity and respect, as well as their right to quality medical care and social services support (People with AIDS Advisory Committee 1983). The media-savvy campaign for rights included calls for attention to the politics and bureaucratic machinations of drug development and to public recognition of women's gender-specific vulnerabilities to infection (Gould 2009; Susser 2009).

The demands made on the medical community and the public writ large ultimately culminated in many productive research alliances. Qualitative health researchers such as Douglas Feldman, Nancy Stoller, Richard Parker, Paul Farmer, Paula Treichler, and Brooke Schoepf began exploring the role of social and political context in understanding HIV infection (see Farmer, Connors, and Simmons 1996 for an impressive review of early literature). Yet even amid growing attention to specific conditions of heterosexual transmission and infection among women, it wasn't until 1987 that *U.S. News & World Report* publicly broke the story that heterosexual individuals who abstain from illicit drug use were potentially at risk for infection too. The disease of the "other," in very specific ways, had finally become a disease of "us" (Farmer 1996, 4; Treichler 1999).

HIV/AIDS Affects Us All

By 1991 HIV/AIDS had become somewhat familiar to many Americans as "an equal opportunity disease" capable of crossing social boundaries of sexuality, nationality, race, class, and gender. At this time AIDS was the leading cause of death among women aged twenty-five to forty-four years in fifteen of the largest U.S. cities (Selik, Chu, and Buehler 1993). Reflecting the increased recognition of HIV in women and heterosexual men and a general sense of alarm about the possible spread of the virus into the American mainstream public, popular media began depicting "the face of AIDS" as heterosexual, female, and middle class (Treichler 1999). Ostensibly the veritable "we" of American culture and society were all at risk. A new kind of urgency fanned the flames of a by now long-standing activist struggle and the public discussion of HIV/AIDS. An intensifying epidemic, mounting activist pressure, and fears concerning the epidemic's future course provided the backdrop against which the Ryan White CARE Act would be adopted and implemented in the United States. Though its particular details were hotly debated in the

House and the Senate, the CARE legislation had broad bipartisan support and passed by a wide margin in the Senate (HRSA 2014a).

The result was a public law providing "disaster assistance" for large urban areas hit hard by the epidemic (Institute of Medicine 2004). The first CARE Act grants were awarded in April 1991 and were administered to state governments and local agencies to fund the building of HIV-related administrative structures and support programs for people living with HIV/AIDS.[2] In that first year CARE Act funding totaled $220.6 million (Institute of Medicine 2004). Including funds for emergency financial relief, end-of-life care, and early intervention, the overarching goal was to provide medical care and palliative and support services for people diagnosed with HIV/AIDS. Education, research, and outreach services were also funded as a means to contain the transmission of HIV. In other words, treatment was part of a prevention strategy.

A key provision in the original 1990 CARE Act legislation stipulated that money had to be dispersed among funding applicants in ways that ensured the money had the "greatest local impact possible" (HRSA 2014a). Thus in the act's early years, resources were spread between states, eligible metropolitan areas (EMAS), and health-related organizations for purposes of capacity-building and services development.[3] Money was annually appropriated and distributed through a formula block grant that calculated funding levels using the number of reported AIDS cases relative to the total population in a given state or EMA (Institute of Medicine 2004). In other words, how much money a given state or EMA was eligible to receive depended on the local prevalence of AIDS. Using AIDS prevalence to determine funding eligibility had the effect of prioritizing states and EMAS with "mature" epidemics rather than areas with emerging epidemics because cases of HIV (not progressed to AIDS) were not counted in the formula (U.S. Congress 2000). In addition Ryan White money was stipulated as "the provider of last resort," meaning that individuals could utilize federally funded HIV/AIDS care programs only if they had no other source of support.

To further ensure the "greatest possible impact" clause in the Ryan White legislation, grant recipients were charged with establishing priorities for the allocation of any funds awarded for an upcoming fiscal year. It required in every case a procedure to obtain community input, whether through the creation of local planning councils or other means (HRSA 2014a). Many communities underwent an annual priority-setting and resource allocation process (for an example, see O'Daniel 2009), whereby HIV-positive individuals, care providers, volunteers, and health professionals worked together to allocate percentages of Ryan White dollars to the various service categories represented in their states and EMAS. This procedure enabled communities to distribute federal dollars prior to their being awarded and according to local needs, which were identified in part through personal experiences with service provision and reception.

Explicit policy language outlined that funding allocations should be based on local conditions and priorities of need. The Ryan White model of funding and care thus presupposed "no one right way to set priorities and allocate resources. . . . Decisions about priorities and allocations should be data-based . . . and consider many different perspectives" (HRSA 2014b). Systems of care therefore unfolded differently in local settings across the country. Large metropolitan areas with well-developed reporting systems and proof of high late-stage disease prevalence clearly received more funds than areas with low late-stage disease prevalence and/or states with underdeveloped epidemiological surveillance structures. Densely populated states and EMAS developed a full range of programmatic services that complimented medical care, including child care, emergency financial assistance, transportation services, hospice care, and acupuncture. Smaller states and/or those with fewer reported AIDS diagnoses developed much more limited systems of care (Marx et al. 1997; Valverde et al. 2004).

The Early Years and Survival

In these early years of the Ryan White CARE Act, the discourse of survival was central to programmatic services in the sense that HIV-infected individuals seldom realized the goal of living long-term with HIV disease. In the 1980s and early 1990s HIV/AIDS was a major cause of death among adults in the United States (HRSA 2014a), and in 1995 the *New York Times* reported it as *the* leading killer of adults aged twenty-five to forty-four.[4] CARE Act funds and programs provided the impetus at this time for increasing the chances that appropriate drugs and services would be developed for populations hit hard by the epidemic and under-served by the traditional health care system.

Given that medical treatment regimens for HIV disease were in their infancy (Zivoudine, or azidothymidine [AZT], was the only treatment available until the Food and Drug Administration [FDA] approved the first protease inhibitor in 1995), official discourses of survival focused on the elaboration of biomedical knowledge of HIV disease. A MEDLINE database search for HIV-related research studies published between 1985 and 1996 highlights the widespread interest in survival as a biomedical and public health phenomenon and goal. The MEDLINE database houses more than three thousand publications for this period, most of which concern topics such as viral incubation (Alcabes, Muñoz, et al. 1993; Ameisen and Capron 1991), cell response (Alcabes, Schoenbaum, and Klein 1993), immunologic profiles and disease progression (Becherer et al. 1990; Buchbinder et al. 1994; Coates et al. 1990; Dickover et al. 1994; Keet et al. 1994), incidence and outcome of opportunistic infec-tion (Bacellar et al. 1994; Centers for Disease Control 1993, 1994), dif-ferential survival with AIDS (Friedland et al. 1991; Lemp et al. 1994; Rothenberg et al. 1987; Turner et al. 1994), and the efficacy of clinical treatment (Fischl et al. 1990; Graham et al. 1992; Koblin et al. 1992).[5] Research trends make clear a logical concern with correlations between epidemiological populations, viral burden, health intervention and/or behaviors, disease progression, and mortality. The novelty of HIV dis-ease meant that the scientific and public health response to the epidemic necessarily concentrated on the basic science of the virus. Slowing the advance of AIDS meant first understanding the cause of the disease and then what happens in the times between HIV infection, illness, and death (Barnett and Whiteside 2002, 32). The term "survival," in this sense, was public health language referring to the proportion of HIV-positive individuals who lived a defined period of time.

Just five years later, however, new conditions circumscribing "sur-vival" would change the meanings and uses of the term in many ways. In 1996 the first protease inhibitors were born, and, with them, highly active antiretroviral therapy (HAART). Across the country HIV/AIDS phy-sicians were reeducated to hit HIV hard and early while using HAART, as it was the new standard of care. For this reason 1996 is recognized as a pivotal year in the public health battle against HIV/AIDS. The existence of the medications themselves was momentous, yet it was the amendment and reauthorization of the CARE Act in that same year that brought the medication, and thus new conditions of survival, to the masses.

Reauthorizing the Ryan White CARE Act,
Rethinking Survival

The 1996 reauthorization bill extended the life of the Ryan White CARE Act until 2000. Several changes in the bill ensured that CARE Act funds would continue to have the greatest impact possible in the era of HAART. Perhaps the most important change for CARE Act programmatic service users was the new funding accommodations for the AIDS Drug Assistance Program (ADAP), or the major mechanism by which people living with HIV disease receive free medication. ADAP became a separate line item under Title II of the act, largely because of the proven effectiveness of HAART and the increased programmatic service enrollment rates.[6] At this time the federal Ryan White budget grew from the initial $220.6 million in 1990 to $738.5 million in 1996 and $996.3 million in 1997 (Institute of Medicine 2004). Sixty-five percent of the 1997 increase went to ADAP. States and EMAS continued to control the distribution of funds among various service categories covered by Ryan White legislation, but it was clear that ADAP was a top priority for all. For example, in many states, funds for hospice services were increasingly redistributed to other services because more HIV-positive people were living with the virus than dying from the disease (Young et al. 2003).

In a very short time frame, many HIV-positive Americans had recovered or maintained their health with the help of HAART (Levine et al. 2007). Calculations concerning survival with HIV disease began to reflect more clearly defined longitudinal terms, as it could now be measured by months *or* years and correlated with blood work that quantified the number of CD4 cells and the number of human immunodeficiency virus copies found in a milliliter of an infected individual's blood. Although CD4 cell counts had been tracked among HIV-positive patients since the late 1980s (Epstein 1996), the FDA's approval of antiretroviral treatment regimens and viral load quantification techniques in 1996 lent new meaning to CD4 cell tracking. Statistical epidemiologists had long been able to correlate declining numbers of CD4 cells to AIDS-defining opportunistic infections and impending death (Corbett 2009, 112; Epstein 1996; Keating and Cambrioso 2003). However, in the context of antiretroviral therapeutic management, changes in CD4 cell counts, when viewed in relation to viral load, were now used to assess the efficacy of treatment regimens. Physicians and patients henceforth had the ability to gauge treatment response and medication adherence, to predict longer-term health, and to prevent disease progression.

In pragmatic terms, technologies of HIV health have enabled improved survival rates, advances in population health, and better quality of life for many people living with HIV disease. These gains are indeed legacies of the Ryan White CARE Act insofar as it provided the impetus for drug development and health care systems elaboration. To the credit of HIV/AIDS "veterans," activists and advocates, researchers, and legislative allies who fought for the act, AIDS-related deaths declined in the United States by 47 percent between 1996 and 1997 (HRSA 2014a). The development of HIV medical treatment options, sophisticated drug regimens, and a better understanding of HIV progression in the human body led to a general decline in AIDS-related death. Simply put, HIV/AIDS was, for many people, no longer the death sentence it once seemed to be.

In this context of increasing trends toward long-term survivorship, of a changing epidemiological landscape, and of successful and expanding Ryan White programmatic services, the discourse of HIV survival further shifted. In Midway and beyond, people living with HIV and their allies began reclaiming their lives and "living well with HIV" by engaging in ordinary routines and living fruitfully. In the HAART era, popular and specialty media depicting stories of survival and triumph over HIV/AIDS such as the magazine *poz*, the novel *What Looks Like Crazy on an Ordinary Day* (Cleage 1997), the Showtime television series *Queer as Folk*, the series *Noah's Arc* on Logo TV, and the Broadway sensation *Rent* celebrated the lives and resilience of a first generation of long-term HIV/AIDS survivors. Here before the American people were examples of HIV-positive individuals engaged in the business of living life. *poz* magazine features stories of daily life and survival, even finding banality, irony, and humor in the condition of being HIV-positive. HIV-positive people in the media lived, loved, laughed, and, as was increasingly portrayed, *worked*. Life with HIV was life nonetheless. Thus HIV survival, it seemed, had a new connotation—one beyond "the bare fact" of continuing to live (Comaroff 2007).

It is by now easy to find uses of slogans and imperatives such as "Live well with HIV." They compose the predominant message in contemporary public health campaigns, HIV-related cyberspace, and HIV-related media programming. Public health messages prompt people to consider HIV/AIDS as a chronic (though infectious) disease made manageable by medical science and a life healthfully lived. This understanding of HIV as a manageable and chronic disease, in many ways, represented an effort to contradict stereotypes and myths historically used to stigmatize and discriminate against HIV-positive people. And while it continues to represent the effort to persuade individuals at risk for infection to be tested and know their status, the message makes clear that HIV infection does not preclude quality of life.

However, this pivotal moment in public health unfolded as HIV infection rates and progression to AIDS began to rise steeply among African Americans (Levine et al. 2007). By 1998 approximately half of all males and four-fifths of all females living with HIV/AIDS in the United States were people of color (Parada 2000, 9). African American women, although only 13 percent of the U.S. female population, constituted 53 percent of all AIDS cases among females (Whitehead 1997, 412). In other words, it was predominately among relatively more affluent White populations that HIV/AIDS-related mortality began to decline. While the advent of HAART ushered in the decline of opportunistic infections and AIDS-related mortality among Whites, African Americans experienced a concurrent 40 percent increase in the incidence of opportunistic infection (Parada 2000, 10).

Citing sobering statistics of infection and AIDS-related mortality in communities of color across the nation, the Congressional Black Caucus developed a call to action and requested that President Bill Clinton declare HIV/AIDS a "state of emergency" in racial and ethnic minority communities.[7] In October 1998 HIV/AIDS was underwhelmingly declared a severe and ongoing health crisis in minority communities. Congress shortly thereafter funded the Minority AIDS Initiative as a means of bolstering HIV-related public health programs in communities of color. Despite a $156 million investment in the initiative's efforts to strengthen responses to the epidemic in communities of color, care providers and women living with HIV/AIDS faced a formidable policy obstacle perhaps few foresaw.

The Changing Face of AIDS: The Others of Welfare Reform

At the same time that Congress began to scale up HIV/AIDS programming in communities of color, it also began to scale back a suite of federal antipoverty programs. The retrenchment of U.S. antipoverty programs in some ways began in the 1970s with the Jimmy Carter administration's domestic budget cutbacks (di Leonardo 2008, 4), but it began ascending in earnest via the fiscally austere policies and practices characteristic of the Ronald Reagan–Margaret Thatcher era (Harvey 2005). During this time poverty among African Americans was depoliticized as a civil rights concern and reinterpreted as a problem of culture, immorality, and individual failure (Goode and Maskovsky 2001). Oscar Lewis's (1959) "culture of poverty" thesis had proven hearty in the sense that it was difficult to dispel in popular and social scientific discourse, having been reproduced by Michael Harrington (1962) in *The Other America: Poverty in the United States* and widely adopted for use in Lyndon B. Johnson's War on Poverty. The culture of poverty thesis explained that conditions of poverty generate cultural adaptations and social institutions that are ultimately incompatible with upward mobility. Although critiqued by many social scientists (Goode 2002b; Leacock 1971; Ryan 1976), the thesis was revived in the Reagan-Thatcher era and used as a basis for blaming the "culture of the poor" for the conditions in which they lived.[8] The culminating idea that disproportionately impoverished populations such as African Americans were trapped in a vicious cycle of poverty perpetuated by *their* culture ultimately reinforced a historically driven sense of "otherness" in relation to an American mainstream public. It also obscured policy mechanisms and informal practices by which African Americans were historically and systematically excluded from wealth-generating opportunities in post–World War II America. The exclusion of African

Americans from federal housing subsidies and economic resources through which many White Americans accrued wealth in the years following the Great Depression and the postwar economic boom are still not recognized in popular debates concerning disproportionate rates of impoverishment among African Americans (Henry 2004; Quadagno 1994).

Thus when Ronald Reagan gave his famous 1976 stump speech insinuating that welfare recipients were morally suspect, many Americans accepted his assertions as reasonable. The long-standing and negative association of welfare with racial minority women provided the backdrop against which Reagan asserted that abuse of the welfare system was rampant and that the tax dollars of "hard-working" (presumably White) Americans paid for the lavish lifestyles of social and moral others (Quadagno 1994; Reese 2005, 21–32). Reagan illustrated his assertions with an astonishing case of welfare fraud: "In Chicago they found a woman who holds the record [for fraud]. She used 80 names, 30 addresses, 15 telephone numbers to collect food stamps, Social Security, veterans' benefits for four nonexistent deceased veteran husbands, as well as welfare. Her tax-free cash income alone has been running $150,000 a year" (cited in Prasad 2006, 86).

Throughout his campaign, Reagan painted a vivid and racialized portrait of poverty and moral ineptitude that many Americans held in contempt. Reagan's stump speech resonated with working-class White Americans in part because it tapped into a broader White backlash against civil rights gains and the in-migration of racial minorities across the United States (Reese 2005, 22), as well as a historically driven gendered stereotype of Blackness that depicted Black women as pathological and immoral (Davis 2006, 41; Seccombe 1998). Put simply Reagan did not create this discourse; he tapped into existing social divisions and stereotypes (Prasad 2006). But by obscuring structural inequities driven by racism, gender subordination, and capitalist expansion, Reagan was able to reinforce historically given societal divisions that would pave the way for intensified national social and economic reform. Once in office, Reagan began the process of righting the supposed wrongs of the welfare system by reducing spending for social programs such as the Section 8 housing voucher program, Aid to Families with Dependent

Children, and school lunch programs (Palmer and Sawhill 1982; Stoez and Karger 1990).

Cuts to social spending gained momentum well into the 1990s and persisted into the 2000s. During this time the American political and economic landscape shifted broadly in response to the profit-making needs of corporate capitalism and the resulting transition to a market-based style of governance. Economic globalization gave rise to the deindustrialization of American urban centers (Bourgois 1996; Newman 1994; Piven 2001; Sassen 1996), the subsequent outsourcing of manufacturing work (Di Leonardo 2008; Goode and Maskovsky 2001), the privatization of government assets and services (Horton 2006; Maskovsky 2000; Rylko-Bauer and Farmer 2002), and a process of steady disinvestment in social safety net programs (Goode 2002a; Kingfisher and Goldsmith 2001; Morgen and Maskovsky 2003; Mullings 2001). African Americans also during this time witnessed the mass incarceration of young men in their communities as a result of a racially inflected war on drugs and a burgeoning and increasingly privatized prison industry (Buck 1994; Chien, Connors, and Fox 2000; Mullings 2001). The end result of this shift has been a steep rise in unemployment and deepening poverty in urban communities and communities of color and a widening gap between the wealthy and the poor more generally (Galster, Mincy, and Tobin 2004; Goode and Maskovsky 2001).

The material developments associated with the American transition to a market-based style of governance were also accompanied by the concomitant rise of market-friendly values. In the United States a belief in the free market as a social cure-all that is capable of restoring the promise of American prosperity has given increased import to the notion of "deservingness" (Davis 2004; Goode and Maskovsky 2001; Kingfisher 2001). Deservingness is by now a ubiquitous concept in American political discourse that more recently explains life circumstances and living conditions in terms of wise decision making and moral accountability. In other words, people choose their own destinies, living conditions, and life circumstances. Thus people who deserve to live well and experience upward social mobility are presumably people who work hard and take personal responsibility for their lives by following mainstream moral codes and predominant social values.

The notion of personal responsibility was codified into law with the passage of the 1996 Personal Responsibility and Work Opportunity Reconciliation Act (PRWORA), which intensified the decades-long transformation of the American social safety net by further cutting spending for antipoverty programs. Under the ideological guise of "rational choice," "free will," and entrepreneurship, welfare reform restricted eligibility for state support (Goode and Maskovsky 2001). Specifically PRWORA replaced Aid to Families with Dependent Children with Temporary Assistance to Needy Families, a programmatic service change that essentially decoupled cash assistance from Medicaid enrollment, eliminated the *entitlement* to cash assistance, limited lifetime eligibility to five years, and mandated that recipients work in exchange for their benefits after two years of enrollment (Good and Maskovsky 2001; Lehman and Danziger 2004, 606; Morgan and Weigt 2001; O'Daniel 2009). Harkening back to the culture of poverty thesis and the neoconservative language of the Reagan era, pro-reform legislators garnered support for these changes by arguing that the welfare system promoted "parasitic" behavior insofar as indefinite financial support hindered the development of personal capacities to realize proper morality and economic productivity (Kingfisher 2002, 25). This equation of morality with economic productivity resonated with popularized "welfare queen" imagery, publicly positioning poor women of color as enabled others who manipulate the system simply (and wantonly) because they can. In a deft rhetorical move, welfare had once again been cast as the problem while social inequality had been pushed to the periphery of the public antipoverty discussion. Black women who received welfare, in turn, had been reiterated as pathological subjects in need of behavioral intervention. Many at this time imagined welfare reform as the only suitable means through which the U.S. government could "liberate" poor women from the poverty and social ineptitude that the welfare state was envisioned to have produced.

Moving women off of welfare was for these reasons touted as smart economic and social policy that freed the federal government from wasteful spending (Kingfisher and Goldsmith 2001). The mandate to work was further exalted as a means for instilling values of personal responsibility in women who were presumed to be lacking virtues of honest living (Lehman and Danziger 2004). In actuality, however, the mandate to work in exchange for welfare benefits increased competition for low-skill work by incorporating welfare recipients into the paid labor force (Danziger and Lin 2000; Goode 2002a). This shift had the effect of lowering workers' wages because the low-skill employment market was saturated with unemployed laborers. Conditions of low-wage work and workfare programs consequently deteriorated (Collins 2008; Henrici 2002; Piven 1998). As a result women struggled with intensifying conditions of poverty and social vulnerability.

The economic instability and social marginality that welfare reform produced ultimately exacerbated poor African American women's vulnerability to HIV infection and progression to AIDS by further weakening pathways of access to health care, self-determination, and decision-making power (Gollub 1999; Hays 2003; O'Daniel 2009, 2011). Across the country low-income and impoverished women made tough choices concerning everyday needs and longer-term health risks such as HIV infection (Connors 1996, 93). In some cases, sex work, condomless sex, and needle sharing provided survival strategies by which vulnerable women could attain what they needed (Connors 1992; Fullilove et al. 1990; Koester and Schwartz 1993; Sobo 1999; Sterk 1999). Under circumstances of poverty and inequality, African American women found themselves at increased risk for HIV infection, progression to AIDS, and AIDS-related mortality relative to their White counterparts (Farmer 1996, 23; Lane et al. 2004; Worth 1989). This outcome has been especially challenging in southern states, where local systems and practices of HIV/AIDS care and prevention were not yet well developed.

Transforming the Ryan White CARE Act, Transforming Survival

By the time the Ryan White CARE Act was up again for reauthorization and amendment in 2006, the effects of welfare reform were becoming more clearly visible. The HIV/AIDS epidemic had reached nearly catastrophic proportions in the southern states. In 2002 44 percent of all new HIV infections in the United States were in the southern states (Kaiser Family Foundation 2006), and African Americans constituted 73 percent of all reported HIV/AIDS cases in the region (Fullilove 2006, 11).

By 2004 North Carolina was one of the fifteen states with the highest numbers of African Americans living with HIV; African Americans contracted more than 69 percent of all new HIV infections there. Of those cases 24.5 percent were among African American women (Kaiser Family Foundation 2006), a new generation that was just beginning to reach lifetime eligibility limits for welfare services. And because the South had few densely populated EMAS and historically low AIDS prevalence rates, local systems of care were underfunded and ill-equipped to handle the chronic and intensive service needs of this public health population.

As the epidemic gained momentum in the South and among African Americans living in poverty, public discourse of HIV/AIDS in "Black America" became more prevalent. For example, in 2006 both PBS's *Frontline* and ABC News's *Primetime* showcased stories of the growing epidemic among African Americans in various communities around the country that were poorly equipped to meet their needs. The association of long-standing civil rights concerns and issues such as poverty, residential segregation, and the mass incarceration of Black men with the proliferating HIV/AIDS epidemic were elaborated in the national media limelight. Pointed program titles and media headlines such as "Out of Control: AIDS in Black America" and "NAACP [National Association for the Advancement of Colored People] Leaders Take HIV Test, Call for National Black AIDS Mobilization" helped to leverage popular support for a fiscal expansion of the already burgeoning system of Ryan White CARE programs.

In addition a federally contracted independent assessment of the formula used to determine levels of need in the states and EMAS found that an enhanced formula could take into account relative disease burden and a ranking of need across jurisdictions. This meant that the federal government could potentially consider the maturity of an area's epidemic as well as the severity of need in the area. The committee recommended against the continued use of the existing formula because it benefited EMAS more than it did the states (Institute of Medicine 2004, 3). This advantage partially explained why southeastern states like North Carolina struggled to develop effective reporting systems and structures of care even in the midst of this public health crisis. Taking HIV cases and severity of need into account, the committee surmised, would help to redirect funds to areas of emerging and greatest need. Yet the question of how and whether to amend the Ryan White CARE Act was mired in political controversy.

Activists, allies, and legislators in EMAS with extensive (and expensive) systems of care and histories of advantage in the Ryan White CARE Act's context worried that formula revisions would shrink the absolute dollar amounts made available to them. Fearing a decline in services and a possible reversion in the progress made toward HIV prevention and HIV health recovery and maintenance, EMAS advocated for increasing overall Ryan White funding rather than simply redistributing funds to the South. The months leading up to the 2006 reauthorization were a time of intense discussion and local uncertainty and fear. For example, Jeremy vividly remembered the 2006 reauthorization debates as "scary," "unpredictable," and "intense." Stopping short of characterizing his visits to "the [Capitol] Hill" between representatives of EMAS and elected representatives of southern states as conflict ridden, Jeremy explained how tense the discussions concerning revisions to the formula decision were.

If you looked at areas [cities around here] and how it was playing out at the time, you had a pandemic that was catastrophic, not unlike a third world country minus the infrastructure that we saw in, like, big cities like San Francisco, New York, LA. And the question first was, will the act even be renewed? If so, will it be a photocopy of the original or will it be part of that? So initially this was southern rural versus urban. . . . If you remember, the big proponents of it were Ted Kennedy, Hillary Clinton, . . . and Richard Burr was advocating—he was a senator from Alabama. They were our real champions, saying, "We've got a real problem in the South going on, and you're focused on urban areas and not on rural parts of the country or southern parts in general." So the whole dialogue was heating up and extending so long that we were operating on continuing resolution, continuing resolution. We began to fear that they weren't going to renew the act all because there seemed to be no good answer. So providers were going, "What's going to happen? What are we going to do?" It was truly frightening.

At "the eleventh hour," Jeremy explained, word came through the North Carolina State consortium that the Ryan White CARE Act had been reauthorized in amended form. From his position as an invited speaker at North Carolina's commemoration of World AIDS Day, he was proud to tell the crowd that the Ryan White CARE Act had been reauthorized and changed to better meet the needs of southern states in the midst of this mounting crisis.

The 2006 Ryan White HIV/AIDS Treatment Modernization Act (TMA) defined funding need by the new formula. EMAS that stood to potentially lose federal dollars using the new formula were "held harmless," meaning that they would not receive formula awards less than a specified percentage of what they had received in the base year. In other words, they were ensured at least a specific proportion of their past funding (typically starting at 100 percent the first year and then gradually declining to 92.5 percent in year 3) (National Health Policy Forum 2010). Because of these developments, Ryan White CARE Act funding continued to reach unprecedented levels.

The act was reauthorized for $528 million in 2000 and reauthorized for an additional $264 million in 2006 (HRSA 2014a). This 50 percent increase reflected goals to expand the act's impact across the southern states and to "hold harmless" the promises and enrollment growth due to long-term survivorship and the increasing need for a provider of last resort. In these specific ways, the 2006 TMA was responsive to changing conditions of the epidemic. Under the redefinition of geographic priorities, North Carolina received $6.5 million more in federal funds for fiscal year 2007 than it had in the previous fiscal year. Increased funding in the South thus reflected a careful redirection of funding to "areas of greatest need" and was touted as further evidence of growth in HIV-related public health programs (Office of the Press Secretary 2006).

At the same time, however, the TMA reflected the shift toward a market-based model and ideology of U.S. governance. Specifically the TMA restricted access to programmatic services and decreased funding for antipoverty measures that had been long embedded in the Ryan White CARE Act legislation. Funding advancements for the southern states were therefore implemented alongside two major changes in the legislation, both of which had the effect of further promoting a shift in thinking about and experiencing survival with HIV disease.

First the TMA mandated that 75 percent of all Ryan White CARE Act funds be used on what was considered as "core medical services": outpatient and ambulatory health services, oral health care, and AIDS pharmaceutical assistance. They also included behavioral change programs such as treatment adherence counseling, substance abuse services, and mental health care (USDHHS 2009b). Conversely, funding for support services such as case management, transportation, pastoral care, and emergency financial assistance had to be limited to 25 percent of the funding total. For the first time in the act's history, local priorities of need were subsumed by a federal mandate to limit percentages of Ryan White money available for nonmedical support services. Put another way, the act restricted antipoverty provisions. It was reinforced by a new mandate requiring documentation of the "last resort" measure for emergency financial assistance, meaning that women had to prove they had applied to three other agencies for help before requesting financial support from Health Partnership.

The second major change outlined in the legislation stipulated laboratory testing as a condition of eligibility for Ryan White–funded services. Laboratory analysis of HIV-infected blood had long been a part of routine care for HIV-positive individuals, with quantification of HIV viral loads and CD4, or t-lymphocyte, cells becoming important prognostic markers for disease prognosis with the emergence of antiretroviral medications in 1996 (Moore, Candlin, and Plum 2001). However, it was not until the 2006 TMA that blood work became a criterion for programmatic services participation. In addition to historical criteria of low-income, uninsured, and/or underinsured status (USDHHS 2009b), new policy pronouncements mandated that all persons receiving federally funded benefits and services through the Ryan White CARE Act had to provide documentation indicating their regular participation in medical care. Proof of regular medical care meant presenting health agencies with two consecutive CD4 cell count laboratory tests no more than six months apart. Recipients thus had to continuously update their laboratory work.

Taken together decreased funding for support services and the bloodwork mandate represent another facet of neoliberalism in America insofar as amendments to the Ryan White CARE Act further shifted the responsibility for conditions of life and health onto individuals living with HIV disease. The 2006 Treatment Modernization Act, in other words, fundamentally changed what it means to care for HIV-positive people and the role of the state in mediating survival with HIV disease. Whereas the goal was once to provide palliative care and indefinite support, it was now support for regaining self-sufficiency via personally responsible behavior and, when possible, employment. As the remaining chapters in this book attest, the 75/25 funding split and the blood-work mandate have together engendered new institutional forms of surveillance, accounting, and accountability. As the executive director of the Health Partnership at the onset of this study, Emily, explained,

> Ryan White is much more medicalized than it was when it started. It's about medical service. It's about medical outcome. It's not about paying the rent. It's not about making sure that utilities stay on. And originally it was. That was really what it was all about. And increasingly it's being moved to make sure that people have medical care, that they stay in medical, that they have access to medication, that they have access to the professionals that make all that happen. People can recover their health and, in some cases and for some unknown length of time, their lives with the right support. The question has in some ways become, do our services help people move forward?

As Emily saw it, the Ryan White CARE Act had become, in some ways, a medical program intractably tethered to social prescriptions. Survival, in turn, had come to be associated more generally with notions concerning the correction and/or restoration of people's lifestyles. In official policy phrasing, the Ryan White "legacy of care" and the "miracle" of future promise for HIV-positive people could be realized through care programs that prompted HIV-positive individuals to "get it together" and claim freedom from the burdens of welfare dependency (see HRSA 2010, 1–9).

Reimagining the Ryan White Act's Legacy

Although the United States is home to arguably the most impressive HIV/AIDS care apparatus in the world, it is not isolable from broader cultural conditions and processes spurring the retrenchment of the American social safety net. As I have broadly outlined here, Ryan White legislation, over time, has been made responsive to medical advancement, changing epidemiological trends, American political contingencies, and material and ideological trends associated with social safety net divestment. Indeed, the now decades-long preservation of such an encompassing public health apparatus in the context of these profound shifts is perhaps nothing short of the public health miracle the Health Resources and Services Administration touts it to be. Yet when we suspend the official discourse and look deeply into African American women's experiences with legislative change in Midway, we illuminate how this legacy of care has reproduced conditions of social exclusion and health care inequality.

2. The Local Landscape of HIV/AIDS Care

We've had a lot of growth in our little system. Now it's made up of different funders, the consortium or whatnot, and all these different kinds of care providers. It's like, "what are you all responsible for?" There's all these people and all these services, and you don't know who does what or why they do it that way. . . . Nobody really knows yet what each other's doing or even whether what rules to follow, whether they be state, or federal, or even agency rules. We're just going with the flow as best we can.

PAULA, a Health Partnership employee

In the immediate aftermath of the 2006 Treatment Modernization Act, Midway's system of HIV/AIDS care grew seemingly overnight. The women in this study suddenly had access to a variety of new health-related services in addition to the many social programs long in place. They were potentially eligible for up to fifteen federally funded social programs, the majority of which were funded by the Ryan White CARE Act and administered through Health Partnership. More than half of them were newly implemented as a result of the 2006 TMA. When asked where they turned for support, most women recited a list of programs administered through Health Partnership rather than having approached family, friends, or other social services. Clearly the agency and its programs were an important presence in their lives.

Health Partnership is located in one of Midway's most economically distressed neighborhoods. At the time of this research, dilapidated houses along with empty buildings, abandoned homes, and the remnants of demolition jobs left long unfinished lined the streets. On any given day, people could be seen walking to and from the corner store, which advertised that food stamps and Women, Infants, and Children (WIC) vouchers were accepted in payment for discounted meats. On pleasant days bus stops in the neighborhood bustled with activity as children and adults alike congregated to catch their rides to full-service grocery stores, shopping centers, and movie theaters in other parts of town. As a shopping destination, this particular neighborhood could offer little other than industrial supplies, high-priced convenience stores, and a few small, locally owned restaurants boasting they sold soul food, country cooking, or "a taste of home." Home-based day care centers, churches, and community-based program offices dotted the neighborhood landscape.

Just beyond this neighborhood lay a recently revitalized greater downtown area. The new downtown concept was based around growth projections among Midway's financial sector, real estate markets, and neighborhood-based corporate retail ventures. Amid relatively quiet lawyers' offices, commercial banks, and consulting firms sat bustling buildings with social service offices, a high-rise housing project, a drop-in center for the homeless, and several drug treatment facilities. The colorful and well-kept building facades of the high-finance private sector provided a stark contrast to the relatively muted exteriors of buildings that housed public programs for low-income populations.

Health Partnership sat approximately a mile from the portion of Main Street associated with the heart of downtown. It had no signs advertising what the organization provided or for whom its services were intended. Agency employees and clients explained to me early in this research that HIV disease was a stigmatized condition amid Midway's Black residents. Women in this study frequently reported that friends and loved ones described the viral infection as "having that shit" or "dying of AIDS." Employees sometimes described how friends and acquaintances "fished" for gossip about who was HIV-positive in their neighborhoods and churches. In one case I watched as a passerby tried to confirm his suspicion that an acquaintance was HIV-positive. He had seen his acquaintance enter the building on several occasions and, one day, simply decided to check it out. Another client mistakenly let him into the building. He promptly approached the front desk, demanding to know the agency's purpose. "Is it AIDS?" he asked. "I got a right to know. I know it's AIDS—look at that ribbon [on the wall]! Oh shit, I can't believe it!" he exclaimed. Meanwhile, a seasoned agency employee calmly (and cryptically) explained that Health Partnership served people with a variety of health conditions and, as a general rule of privacy, did not disclose its purpose to walk-ins. The man left seemingly frustrated that he had not been given an unequivocal answer to his question.

A prohibitive building exterior reinforced Health Partnership's privacy protocol. The building's parking lot was surrounded on all sides by a chain-link fence topped with barbed wire that was locked after business hours to protect the property and building from break-ins and vandalism. Around the front of the building, double doors made of bullet-resistant glass provided the public point of entry. Immediately beyond the glass doors was a small foyer with an electronically locked wooden door that closed off Health Partnership's lobby. A sheet of bullet-resistant glass allowed personnel at the reception desk to see into the foyer. Reception desk personnel buzzed in visitors they recognized as clients or other agency staff, but they kept anyone seeming out of place or nosy in the foyer until a further assessment could be made.

At first Health Partnership seemed to me depressing, even foreboding. I perhaps wrongly interpreted the building's exterior features solely as visual pollution, an unsightly disservice to neighborhood residents and clients of the organization. It quickly became clear, however, that staff and clients alike appreciated the security measures. In addition to protecting the clients' privacy, building security proved a safety precaution. On more than one occasion, physical fights migrated from surrounding homes, into the streets, and onto the sidewalk in front of the organization. Gunfire in a neighboring home prompted a police standoff and Health Partnership's mandatory lockdown for a few hours one afternoon. And a few times Health Partnership employees received threatening phone calls, voice mails, and emails from disgruntled and emotionally distraught clients. Bullet holes in the agency's windows hinted at the complicated dynamics among Health Partnership, neighborhood residents, and Midway's HIV-positive population. At the core of these dynamics were the programmatic services through which Health Partnership distributed financial support and other health-related resources to their clients.

In this chapter I describe Midway's federally funded public HIV/AIDS health care continuum in the post-TMA era. To understand the women's lives and experiences of survival requires familiarity with the various programmatic services and personnel they could have turned to for support. I chose to conduct this research through Health Partnership in part because it was Midway's largest and most comprehensive HIV/AIDS support service provider. As such, it was central to the local public HIV/AIDS care system. It was the *only* organization housing several Ryan White–funded programs under a single roof in a community-based setting, and it was frequently lauded for its "one-stop shopping" and client-centered model of care provision. Because of this arrangement, many in the community esteemed the agency. Physicians, case managers, and HIV-testing counselors referred the newly diagnosed to Health Partnership specifically because it was a central point of access to and retention in the broader programmatic service continuum. However, as this chapter attests, Midway's system was in some ways a cumbersome inventory of programmatic service aims, care provision guidelines, and discretionary strategies.

Under the Ryan White CARE Act, Health Partnership received funds for a variety of programs integral to building a system of care capable of meeting the intensive service needs of impoverished and historically disenfranchised populations. For several years prior to this research, the organization administered emergency financial assistance, nutritional assistance, pastoral care, and the AIDS Drug Assistance Program. The women in this study reported having grown used to agency protocol for requesting rental and utilities assistance, medication support, nutritional supplements, and weekly packets of food. However, when I first arrived in Midway in August 2007, Health Partnership was just beginning to reorganize in response to the TMA-mandated policy changes described in chapter 1.

Until that time two full-time staff and two or three volunteers from local college programs led Health Partnership. Clients generally regarded the volunteers and staff as being "like" them insofar as they tended to be African American, at the time lacked college degrees, and preferred an informal service provision style that respected culturally accepted notions of deference to elders. As Greg, an original staff member, explained, "There wasn't a whole lot of structure. Clients could just come in here and ask for assistance with no appointment necessary. They would get it right there and then. I definitely talked to clients a lot more. I felt like I developed personal relationships with the majority of clients. . . . And, you know, I didn't and still don't really try to scold a client. I definitely try to keep it respectful with the clients for the simple fact that some of these clients are my mother's age."

During these early years of Health Partnership, agency services had seemed relatively uncomplicated. Resources and staff were scarce enough that their entire operation was housed in one room in the basement of neighborhood church. Yet despite its limited programs and resources, Health Partnership had early on proven a crucial social resource for Midway's HIV-positive population. Community members lauded it as a "place where you can be HIV-positive," meaning clients felt comfortable disclosing and discussing their health there. For some of the long-term agency clients in this study, Health Partnership during the early 2000s had served as "*the only place*" where they felt safe being "out" as HIV-positive. The small staff size meant fewer people knew a client's HIV-positive status. Additionally Health Partnership's staff was commended for being caring and dedicated individuals. They were, to sum it up, regarded as people who worked their jobs relatively cheerfully for little pay, with few resources, and with even less recognition.

The agency was also federally designated as a payer of last resort, meaning that when all other sources of support failed, an HIV-positive individual in need could turn to Health Partnership for financial help. The agency became increasingly important to those women who had "timed out" of welfare services and/or had few other places to seek assistance. Thus in its capacity as a safe zone with committed employees and accessible financial resources, Health Partnership was well established prior to the 2006 Treatment Modernization Act as an important institution in the local HIV-positive community. However, the act's implementation ushered in the beginning of unprecedented agency growth.

My first day as a participant-observer at the organization marked the arrival of three new employees. The agency could no longer fit in a single-room office. Along with an employee lunchroom and a restroom, the agency had an office for each staff member in the spacious, if old, building. Over the next few months, it hired seven additional employees to run new—and, in some cases, officially undefined—programs. Thus I witnessed a challenging period when new staff members undertook building rapport with community members, designing programs responsive to community needs, and implementing program protocol in ways compatible with federal fiscal oversight mandates. I also saw for myself the "professionalization" of HIV/AIDS care services in Midway. Observations among new staff were crucial to my understanding of Midway's system of care because these service professionals interpreted, implemented, and enacted the new health care policies (Lipsky 1980).

In total Health Partnership employed eleven service providers: six African American women, two African American men, two White women, and one White man. All employees reported coming from middle-class backgrounds, although some discussed the precarious economic nature of their middle-class status to their being single parents, to having financial debt, and/or to living close to relatives who were living in poverty (see Patillo-McCoy 2000). All employees discussed having close family members or friends who lived in poverty, many of whom struggled with substance use. And some employees had themselves at one time struggled with chemical dependency and/or intimate partner violence. Thus most employees regarded the challenging life circumstances that their clients faced as a familiar landscape but potentially traversable given the right support.

All employees, except for Greg, had special certifications, college degrees, and, in some cases, graduate degrees in addition to their experience and training as HIV/AIDS service providers. The apparent preference for employees to have specialized credentials was, in most cases, state mandated. Much like welfare services in the 1970s and 1980s (Naples 1998), the peer counseling methods that characterized a previous generation of Ryan White CARE Act programs were gradually phased out, and the new model of care prioritized specialized sets of "expert" knowledge concerning disease management instead of "insider" knowledge of palliative care or advocacy needs (O'Daniel 2009). Thus state-level job descriptions in the post-TMA era outlined desirable job candidates in terms of education credentials and, in very few cases, years of experience working in an HIV-positive community. The general trend was that Midway's HIV/AIDS services were being increasingly professional-ized. As a result Health Partnership's newest employees were creden-tialed with degrees and certifications in social work, health education, counseling, divinity, and nutritional science.

The professionalization of Health Partnership staff coincided with the policy emphasis on oversight and behavioral compliance discussed in chapter 1. I want to note here, however, that the employees' educa-tional training and discipline-specific philosophies had previously pre-pared them for the behavior change work undergirding the Treatment Modernization Act. Natasha, for example, explained:

> The codes and ethics of the social work practice are with me every-day. I never understood what they really meant, but I see now the things that I learned as far as keeping boundaries, as far as listening, and the things they taught us to be a good social worker helps me now with these clients. Like, for example, you have to take your whole matter and stop putting on Band-Aids. So I start with the idea that I'm trying to show these clients that case management is not a life-style. It's a stepping-stone. They have to learn to do for themselves. It's just the philosophy that I learned.

Monica similarly explained, "One of the main things you learn about health education is changing behavior. With changing behavior there's a lot of different theories and models you have to use. . . . I try to figure out which one to use or what would be the best one to use. You have to look at certain issues—like, what's their education level, income level—because a lot of things like that affect how a person lives and what they can do about their health."

As Natasha and Monica described, employees interpreted their work as HIV/AIDS service providers through the lenses of their educational training. Their training, like that of their fellow employees, emphasized behavior modification insofar as they equated the need for services with individual deficits in knowledge or motivation. The idea was that clients must be persuaded or taught to change behaviors deleterious to their health. However, employees also drew from a "strengths perspective" focused on positive attributes and skills that clients bring to bear on their health strategies. Positive attributes include health-promoting capacities such as courage, spirituality, intelligence, paid employment, stable housing, and/or social skills (Butler and Smith-McKeever 2003). Employees generally tried to address the unique needs of each individual by identifying behavioral modification needs and drawing on client strengths to promote behavior change.

In addition to their formal training, many Health Partnership employees were personally motivated to work at an HIV/AIDS service organization. Natasha, for example, switched from working at a traditional social work site after learning that a former classmate in her hometown was diagnosed as HIV-positive. For Natasha the realization that "AIDS was that close to me" prompted her to think about the epidemic in community terms. She often discussed HIV disease as a social problem that the Black community should address. Focusing her social work skills on issues of HIV/AIDS became one means for her to address a community need. Most employees similarly felt that given their personal backgrounds, HIV/AIDS care work was an extension of their commitments to community and family. As Ivy put it, "I get up and come to work here everyday because my community needs me to. They are my family." Service providers in this way drew from notions of reciprocity and mutual aid that are often found among African American informal social networks (see Naples 1998; Newman 2001; Stack 1974, 1996). Thus the programs and procedures of this local care continuum were implemented by people with both personal and professional motivations shaping their engagement with federal policy and procedures.

Health Partnership Programs in the Post-TMA Era

Under new conditions of the TMA, Midway's HIV/AIDS system of care continued to include the Emergency Financial Assistance (EFA) Program. Indeed, this particular program was the heart of the agency's operation, even though it was part of the "25 percent" funding category. It was the most sought-after service by clients and was the agency's most expensive program, not including the state-administered ADAP. Funding for the EFA Program was provided through the Housing Opportunities for People with AIDS program (HOPWA) and through Ryan White legislation. Both streams of funding were federal in nature and were specifically designated as payers of last resort. Every dollar was made available to HIV-positive persons in need of cash for monthly rent and utilities.

As a provider of last resort, the emergency component of the funds was supposed to be strictly enforced. Yet as one service provider explained, yearly Ryan White budgets had to be spent in their entirety. Any unspent funds were subtracted from the state budget the following fiscal year; unspent money, in other words, was forever lost to the state of North Carolina. Greg explained, "When I first started, I just kind of had the mentality, like, is it in my budget? I know if I don't spend this money out, we won't get it back for the next fiscal year. So I would just spend, and I would help anybody regardless of the situation if they were showing up here with a need."

Greg's strategy of allocating his money solely on the basis of request changed with the advent of the 75/25 split mandated by the Treatment Modernization Act. In his estimation eligibility procedures had to be tightened to compensate for the new oversight guidelines and the decreased amount of available money for support services. The realities of how the budget worked, however, did not change. Greg still had to spend each month's money in its entirety or lose that money for the next fiscal year. Reimbursement procedures further complicated Greg's operation; Health Partnership had to "float" disbursed funds, often waiting months for reimbursement from the federal government. To reconcile the need to spend, the imperative to spend wisely, and the reality of lagging reimbursement, people applying for assistance were required to prove and *justify* their need.

First, applicants were required to bring in an eviction notice from their landlord or a letter of disconnection from the utility company. Officially it was never entirely clear to agency employees whether such documents and dire circumstances were eligibility conditions mandated by the TMA. Employees informally implemented and strategically used this policy during times when the organization was waiting to be reimbursed for its services by the federal government. In other words, requiring documentation provided one means of prioritizing the distribution of funds when resources were scarce.

In addition Greg strategically prioritized rental assistance applications. Aside from wanting to avoid seeing a client evicted, Greg knew where he could "buy time" for clients. For example, local utility companies granted consumers twenty-one days beyond a bill's due date before disconnecting services. A disconnection notice could thus allow the EFA Program counselor to make a verbal commitment for payment on behalf of the client without having to actually pay for another three weeks. This strategy kept both the clients' power on and Health Partnership from overextending its budget in any single month. The drawback, however, was that clients would often wait until their circumstances were extreme before coming to the organization to discuss their support options. In some cases clients lost power or were evicted because they had been unable to schedule a timely appointment for assistance. In other cases clients were denied support because the organization was on a spending freeze. Thus this strategy of positioning one's self as undeniably in need of care from the provider of last resort could be risky.

The second EFA Program protocol criterion required clients to explain why in that particular month, or months, their income was not enough to meet their needs. For some women, this task was fairly simple. They would attend their appointments with receipts for hospital bills, car repairs, and/or insurance premiums in hand. Nonpayment of rent or utilities could be justified with acceptable unexpected or unavoidable expenses. For example, Taylor found herself unable to pay her rent and utilities one month. She had recently purchased several books for her undergraduate coursework and needed to buy a bus ticket to visit her seriously ill daughter. Before purchasing the ticket, she spoke with the EFA Program counselor to make sure that she was not mistaken in her strategy. Only after being assured that she could get assistance did she go ahead and make the purchase.

Kareese, however, experienced the emergency protocol differently. Kareese scheduled an appointment for emergency assistance when she realized that she had misspent her rent money for the upcoming month. After a particularly stressful day of fighting with her husband, Kareese relapsed and spent her rent money on drugs, alcohol, and expensive new tennis shoes. She returned the tennis shoes the following day but could not undo the fact that she had spent half of her rent money on drugs. Before her scheduled appointment, Kareese confided in me that she was not planning on disclosing where her money had been spent.

Just minutes before her meeting with the EFA Program counselor, she was trying to think of how she might explain her situation without disclosing her drug use. She feared Health Partnership would reject her application because of how she had spent her disability check. In the end, Health Partnership did provide Kareese with the financial support she needed, but she felt that the staff had lectured and shamed her for spending her income in a technically inappropriate way.

Finally clients who requested emergency assistance had to provide proof they attended health care appointments. Proof consisted of up-to-date laboratory printouts indicating the amount of HIV and number of CD4 cells in their bloodstream.[1] Reviewing this laboratory work over time theoretically allowed care providers to assess an applicant's compliance with physician recommendations. To my knowledge few clients were turned away using this assessment technique. Clients seemed to generally understand and follow this rule with little resistance. For clients who did not display favorable health outcomes on their laboratory work, staff provided medication adherence counseling rather than denying them services.

Together these eligibility requirements and employee strategies often meant that a client would come in needing funds for two or three months of rent and/or several months of utilities payments. Whether a client received the full amount requested depended on the funds available, their history of using emergency assistance, and their ability to sway Greg to use his discretion in their favor.[2] Kareese, for example, explained that Greg had given her the assistance she needed because she had been working hard to maintain sobriety and "live right" even though she sometimes "messed up." Indeed, many women in this study who struggled with chemical dependency or other such technically "unacceptable" financial burdens could count on their powers of persuasion to help them out of a financial jam.

Greg was one of the two original members of Health Partnership. His status as "an original" was important to clients who were distrustful of the restrictive changes ushered in by the TMA and the agency's rapid growth. Greg's status also meant that he had known many clients for a number of years, so he was familiar with the trajectories of most clients' housing situations and economic circumstances. More than half of the daily phone calls made to the organization were for Greg. Easily three-quarters of the walk-in clients who went to the organization wanted to see him. When it came to receiving timely and personalized service, he was, in the words of one woman, "the Man."

In addition to EFA Program funds, Health Partnership administered funds designated under the categorical umbrella of "medical case management," which was a new core service implemented as a result of the Treatment Modernization Act. Clients could request assistance with copayments for HIV medication and/or non-HIV-related medications that were approved by Medicaid. Clients could also seek financial support for dental work and copayments for physician appointments. Thus as the medical case manager, Monica served as the distributor of medical case management funds.

Monica's job description also included enrolling clients into the AIDS Drug Assistance Program, which is jointly funded by individual states and the federal government. In North Carolina uninsured HIV-positive individuals who had an income at or below 300 percent of the poverty level qualified for participation in the program. ADAP provides free medications for the treatment of HIV disease in addition to medications for the treatment of opportunistic infections associated with HIV disease. At the time of this research, the ADAP medication list included antiretroviral, antidepressant, anti-lipidemic, antihypertensive, antidiabetic, and antimicrobial medications, to name just a few of the available drug classes. The drugs and drug classes included as ADAP-eligible medications treat ailments and infections that are considered common to individuals with HIV infection (such as metabolic disorders of the liver, diabetes, hypertension, and depression). Monica's job was to help eligible individuals complete the application paperwork for program enrollment.

Monica's other programmatic responsibility was to function for both drug assistance programs as the treatment adherence counselor. Indeed, part of Monica's personally developed criteria for the dispersal of Ryan White medication funds was that clients had to indicate their commitment to and understanding of their medication regimens. This informal requirement of the medical case management program emerged over time in response to Monica's increasingly restrictive monthly budget.

For example, in a typical month Monica could distribute $4,000 of Ryan White money for medication copayments. At roughly $3 per copayment, she could potentially cover a great deal of medications; however, the need for medication assistance consistently outweighed the available resources. Many clients found themselves with copayments for as many as fifteen medications per month. At roughly $45 per month per individual, Monica could help only around eighty-nine applicants out of the roughly three hundred clients the organization served. Likewise, the scarce funds available for dental work and doctor's visits were far exceeded by need. Monica could distribute only around $800 of Ryan White money per month for these needs. At roughly $10 per physician visit and $250 for the average dental visit, this portion of the money was often promised months in advance of the payment.

Despite Monica's budgetary constraints, many women in this study considered her as a close ally of the clients. Her entry point into the community, however, had been as a general case manager at another social service organization that served HIV-positive populations. Her ties to the community were also personal because she lived in Midway among many of the clients whom she served. Her "insider" status gave her a vantage point for understanding the daily stresses and strains that her clients experienced. This appreciation, in turn, gave Monica what she referred to as "a way to come at clients from a place of empathy." Empathy was generally valued as a service provision tool for building and communicating trust with persons in distress.

Leslie, for example, created and implemented Health Partnership's outpatient substance abuse program, which was also designated as a core medical service. The protocol for designing and implementing the substance abuse program, however, was not outlined in the legislation. Per Health Partnership's *organizational* philosophy, individuals could not be denied services based on their drug use habits, their drug use history, or their unwillingness to attend drug cessation programs. While clients were not officially required to attend substance abuse counseling or support groups as a condition of using Health Partnership services, organization employees referred them on several occasions. For example, Lady E. began her road to recovery just as I began this research. For two months before I arrived, she had attended biweekly substance abuse meetings at a local university hospital. Despite Lady E.'s apparent personal commitment to maintaining her sobriety as well as her institutional commitment to the hospital addiction recovery program, Leslie consistently asked her to attend Health Partnership's substance abuse recovery meetings. Leslie felt that Lady E. would be a good role model for others in the program. She also felt that Lady E. would have a better chance of maintaining her sobriety if she were connected to more than one support group. On a few occasions, however, Leslie also commented that she needed to "fill her group out" to ensure future funding for the program. Lady E. was never penalized for her decision not to attend, but she was prompted on several occasions to join the group.

Armed with the official organizational philosophy of empathy and non-judgment in mind, Leslie created Health Partnership's substance abuse program to loosely mirror the traditions of the motivation enhancement technique (MET), a systemic approach to drug addiction therapy. Based on the principles of motivational psychology, the primary goal of MET is to produce rapid, internally motivated change. Engendering this change meant that Leslie endeavored to help illicit drug–using clients decide for themselves that it was time to quit. Leslie primarily applied conversational strategies such as assessing a client's personal risk of illness, death, social ostracism, and financial hardship due to drug use. She further emphasized one's own responsibility for change. She paired these strategies with her empathy, her advice to stop drug use, and the creation of options to produce change.

I joined Leslie and a client named Chantelle one day during an informal conversation about the difficulties of being homeless and chronically ill. Leslie listened intently as Chantelle described the frustrations and obstacles she faced daily for achieving life stability. Leslie acknowledged Chantelle's feeling that she had "got the run around" from service providers who were supposed to help her obtain much-needed identification cards. Leslie further nodded in agreement when the woman discussed the anger and sadness she felt at being treated unfairly by people who were supposed to help her. At the end of the conversation, Leslie responded with, "Wow, that sounds really hard. But let me ask you this: Do you think things would be easier for you if you quit using? I mean, would you be treated different if you didn't use?" Thus began a conversation between Leslie and Chantelle about strategies for changing the role of addiction in her life. Leslie then continued using the MET with Chantelle in a group format in addition to their one-on-one counseling sessions.

As a woman who has traveled the roads of recovery, Leslie worked hard to facilitate shared dialogue with her clients. Her most important tool, she described, was self-disclosure: "And if I'm with women, I'll talk about my sexual past, my personal history, and being in active addiction. Because staying drunk all the time, you get screwed a lot when you don't plan to. People are more comfortable talking to somebody who you think has been there." Self-disclosure, as Leslie so aptly stated, was a strategy for increasing communication and trust between herself and her clients. Although at the time of this research Leslie was a newcomer to Midway's HIV-positive community, her personalized strategies for relationship building provided a means for bridging the gap, so to speak, between herself as the professional care provider and the clients in need of her professional services. Thus as with Greg and Monica's programmatic procedures for financial assistance, Leslie's protocol for outpatient substance abuse counseling services was also drawn from knowledge and trust based in personal circumstances and relationships.

Like its substance abuse program, Health Partnership's risk reduction counseling program was strictly voluntary. The federal program protocol at this time was known as Comprehensive Risk Counseling Services (CRCS), which provided individually oriented risk reduction and intervention service. Risk reduction in this context primarily referred to reducing one's risk of HIV reinfection or transmission, but it was based on a philosophy of self-determination. Clients thus chose which risks they wished to reduce in their lives so long as they could be related to efforts aimed at minimizing one's chances of HIV reinfection and transmission. Social obligations, legal matters, financial obstacles and strategies, drug use behaviors, and sexual behaviors—all could fall under the purview of CRCS. One woman utilized the CRCS program as a stepping-stone for starting her own business. She and the CRCS counselor spent their sessions together writing business plans, figuring out budgets and revenues, and ordering cost-efficient materials for the business. As they completed these business steps, they discussed how financial security and autonomy could also reduce the client's need for and risk of engaging in condomless sex.

Because CRCS required the disclosure of potentially damaging and otherwise sensitive information, trust was paramount between the CRCS counselor and her clients. In North Carolina one's failure to use a condom and/or to notify one's partner of his or her HIV-positive status is in violation of public health laws. The violation is punishable by fines that could reach $300 or more and, as seen periodically on the news, could include incarceration. CRCS was one program where reporting requirements did not include notification to police or other social service agencies. Clients were technically free to speak about practices and behaviors that were considered illegal or as potentially endangering others. Paula, the CRCS counselor, achieved trust with her clients by maintaining a service provision philosophy based in strategies for building trust while maintaining distance and communicating empathy. Paula's professional demeanor paradoxically relied upon connoting caring and compassion while making it clear that she does not care enough about a person's personal habits to breach confidentiality and "tell their business" to others. As Paula described, "I don't really care too much who it is but what you are doing, and getting into the frame where I know this is personal. And I don't care. Like I care to a certain extent, but I don't. Not enough to put your business out there, you know. But it's about being real and being there for them, to give them whatever that they need to fill that void."

Paula's service provision style, while certainly different from Leslie's protocol of self-disclosure, lent a particular type of formality to her program. This formality, in turn, created a programmatic structure that felt conceptually distinct from the more informal dynamics favored by the EFA Program and the substance abuse program counselors. Clients who needed someone to whom they might safely disclose sensitive information appreciated Paula's strategy of maintaining "professional distance." Thus while all of Health Partnership's programs and procedures were housed under one roof, "the feel" and strategies of different programs varied.

Of all the federally funded AIDS care programs at Health Partnership, nonmedical case management was known among the women in this study as the most rigidly and systematically implemented. Under Ryan White legislation, nonmedical case management provided assistance for a variety of needs that were not directly health related. While a case manager may have given clients advice and assistance in choosing a doctor, they did not follow up on medical appointments, diagnoses, and treatment regimens prescribed by physicians. Nonmedical case managers most often focused on helping clients who had needs that were social, legal, and/or financial in nature.

As a support service, nonmedical case management relied on funds that were part of the 25 percent split to pay case manager salaries and to keep the programs running. "Support service" status meant that case managers had to be perhaps more mindful of federal budgetary constraints and oversight mandates. While case managers did have the discretion to distribute EFA Program funds, clients tended to see program guidelines as more rigid and less likely to pay out without a hassle. In many cases the women opted to wait several days for an appointment with Greg rather than scheduling an appointment with either Bert or Natasha, the agency's case managers. Thus Greg was frequently overbooked. If the clients had waited for "emergency status," then they usually had to schedule the appointment with a different case manager.

When asked to describe the hassle of using case management, however, many women referred to the case managers' styles of providing services rather than to the institutional rules. In the agency context Ryan White–funded case management was largely a referral service aimed at increasing access to health care and related programs. As professionally trained social workers and health care educators, case managers were the primary points of contact between clients and other programs within the system of care, including medical services. Case managers facilitated the clients' enrollment in social programs, their greater understanding of HIV disease, and their empowerment to take responsibility for their health and their daily life circumstances. Empowerment was theoretically achieved when a client maintained her health care regimen and finances with little or no support from programmatic service representatives. However, according to Natasha, assisting a client achieve full empowerment had not yet happened in her career. Still with fostering clients' empowerment to produce their own good health outcomes as an ultimate programmatic goal, case management was implemented as a short-term program. As Natasha described it, "Case management is only there to help you from where you are diagnosed. If you are newly diagnosed then you maybe need to get medical services, nutrition, housing. We help you get all that established by connecting you with Medicaid, applying for Social Security—as far as appeals and denials—looking at housing, finding food. But after a certain amount of time, with all that established, then what is there a need for us to do?"

Natasha described how the goals of case management could be achieved through service enrollment. Bert, however, explained the other component of case management: "All of the things about finances, household, and medical care are very important. But you can look at it like, how does the person keep their appointments? How responsible are they when it comes down to appointments, if that's their concerns, or are they just concerned about getting their rent paid now? The most important thing is your health, and if you're not in compliance with that, it's really not no need for me to help you. You will be sick anyway."

Bert's explanation of assessing a client's progress within the case management program underscored the strategic need for clients to communicate an earnest desire to achieve health empowerment as a condition of eligibility. Meeting this condition meant that much like contemporary welfare programs, the utilization of HIV/AIDS care services as previously described was theoretically a temporary measure. Over time clients should be "hooked into the system" securely enough to navigate their own way through medical care and daily life with HIV disease. Clients reported feeling as though case managers did not trust them because they asked a lot of questions about current circumstances and potential strategies for avoiding such circumstances in the future.

In addition to housing emergency-based and temporary programs, Health Partnership administered long-term programs that were funded through means other than the Ryan White CARE Act. These programs included a weekly food pantry, a nutritional assessment service, and a pastoral care program. These services were not Ryan White funded at the time of this research, although agency administrators thought it likely that nutritional assessments would receive such funds in the future. Individual donations, agency fund-raisers, the State Nutritional Assistance Program, and the Federal Emergency Management Agency funded the food pantry.[3] Each client who complied with the state HIV/AIDS consortium's annual update policy was eligible to "shop" the food pantry once weekly for approximately fifteen to twenty-five items. Each client received one protein item, such as frozen hamburger meat or frozen chicken, in addition to whatever fresh produce and canned goods had been donated or were available at the food bank's distribution center that week. Although the pantry's inventory varied greatly from week to week, clients could generally count on several nutritious, if sometimes less than mouth-watering, choices.

The pastoral care program was one of the founding programs of the agency. In past years pastoral care had been legislatively considered as psychosocial support and thus as part of Ryan White CARE Act programs. The implementation of the TMA ushered in new definitions of psychosocial support that did not include pastoral care, so the agency paid for this program through its fund-raising efforts. It was, in other words, an agency-sponsored service. Any client wanting to speak with the pastoral care counselor could do so at any time. Doug, Midway's pastoral care counselor, was an eager listener who worked hard to maintain good working relationships with clients. He accepted walk-in appointments and prescheduled appointments alike. He made house calls when necessary and prided himself on being a patient and active listener. In addition to serving as a faith-based, nonemergency counselor, Doug matched clients with local "care teams," which usually consisted of several members from an area church congregation who wanted to provide spiritual support and companionship for a person living with HIV/AIDS. While this particular program did not receive federal funding and did not have the relatively large budgets of other services, it nonetheless served as an important component in many women's experiences with the system of HIV/AIDS care.

Lisa, for example, spoke informally with Doug on a regular basis. At the time of this research she did not have a care team. Lisa had participated in the program in the past and had recently attended an agency-affiliated spiritual retreat for HIV-positive individuals. One afternoon Lisa and I talked privately in a conference room at Health Partnership. She was "unnerved" by a series of dreams that she characterized as being suicidal. In her dreams, Lisa jumped off a mountainside but always awoke before she hit the ground. She discussed how she awoke from the dreams feeling anxious and confused but not exactly afraid. Lisa also often said how lucky she felt to be alive and wondered why she kept having the dreams even though she did not feel as though she wanted to hurt herself. The dreams occupied her thoughts and made her uncomfortable. She decided to talk to Doug about the dreams and see if he had any insights as to how serious they might be. Doug had known Lisa for several years and was confident that she was not suicidal. He talked with Lisa about the spiritual symbolism of cliff jumping. He suggested that Lisa's recent attendance at the spiritual retreat was a "jumping-off point" for a new spiritual journey. He advised her to view the jump in metaphorical rather than suicidal terms. This advice calmed Lisa's fears that she might be unconsciously suicidal and provided her with an alternative means for understanding an otherwise unsettling series of dreams and thoughts. Thus although Lisa might not consistently participate in Health Partnership's pastoral care services, they represented an important health resource to which she turned as needed.

The eight services at Health Partnership were designed to operate together as a safety net for individuals who were in danger of dropping out of medical care or were experiencing interruptions in medication adherence. While Ryan White–funded programs represent one of the largest public health efforts in American history, they do not operate in isolation; rather, the system of HIV/AIDS support services and medical care articulates with other federal social programs. The institutional context of the study participants' lives thus included several other programs and policies that dramatically affected their abilities to care for themselves and their health.

Beyond the Purview of the Ryan White CARE Act

In addition to HIV/AIDS support services and more commonly known welfare services such as WIC and Temporary Assistance to Needy Families (TANF), the women in this study drew support from myriad other social programs. The Social Security Disability Insurance (SSDI) and Supplemental Security Insurance (SSI) programs provided the backbone of many HIV-positive women's income-generating strategies.[4] Monthly disability insurance payments were an important means of income and provided access to other related support services such as subsidized bus passes and other forms of transportation assistance. The women who qualified for disability insurance payments based on their HIV-positive status also had to meet two health criteria: they had to have been diagnosed with AIDS and had to have experienced at least two opportunistic infections since their diagnosis with HIV/AIDS. Many women who felt physically and/or emotionally sick due to HIV disease sought disability status. It was also a goal for women who reported no illness symptoms but had few other options for finding steady income.

Monthly disability payments ranged from $623 to more than $1,000, based on one's work history and the cumulative amount of money one paid in Social Security taxes. From a service provider standpoint, making ends meet on a disability income was a difficult road, so to speak, that should be avoided. Greg explained why he counseled clients not to enroll in disability benefits programs: "This is what you guys have agreed to live on for the rest of your lives. I don't know why they would wait around for two or three years to collect disability when they know they don't have that much of a work history. Their disability check is going to be five hundred a month, and it'll be like that for rest of their lives because you haven't put into the system."

Greg explained that monthly disability incomes can be meager. His point that gaining disability status would not solve women's economic problems was generally well taken. Yet the women's decisions to apply for and receive disability payments reflected much more than the "waiting to collect" mentality that Greg described as central to the women's decisions to use the program. Enrollment in the disability income program reflected a variety of factors and daily life conditions other than their health. The reality was that finding and keeping a job was no simple task. Disease symptoms, depression, a history of incarceration, mental health issues, and drug addiction—all shaped the women's abilities to compete in the local job market. The reality for many women was that they were unable to find full-time, well-paying employment. Disability income was thus sometimes seen as a luxury by women who did not qualify for it and who endeavored to find stable, well-paying employment. Marjorie, for example, struggled to feed herself and her two young sons on income generated from part-time, insecure work. Marjorie attended a free culinary school program in the afternoons and then sought work as a day laborer after her courses each day. She often found work in construction and construction site maintenance. This work was sporadic at best and physically taxing. Although Marjorie was in good physical health, she found it physically and emotionally draining to attend classes in the morning, perform manual labor in the afternoons, and then care for her children in the evenings.

On several occasions Marjorie came into Health Partnership sweaty, rushed, and out of breath. She hurried to the organization during her lunch break at work so she would not miss being able to shop at the food pantry. More times than not she came in "hot," or angry, because she felt that she was physically working harder than the men around her did. She could not quit this work, however, because it was all she could find that would grant her the flexibility she needed to care for her children (one of whom suffered from a chronic kidney disease) and to attend school.

Throughout the course of this study, Marjorie struggled to make ends meet on a monthly basis, sometimes earning as little as $200 a month. The difficulties of paying monthly bills through part-time, insecure work were exacerbated by her disqualification from welfare cash assistance services. After the birth of her first child, Marjorie's boyfriend was released from prison. He had plans to move in with Marjorie and help her with the baby. They were keeping their plans secret so as not to alert welfare officials that an aid recipient was living with a convicted felon. Upon his release, he was required to provide address verification. Unfortunately for Marjorie, he gave the Department of Corrections her address without realizing the consequences. As she explained,

> Just by him putting my address on there—I don't know what Social Services had to do with this, but I think it might have been for his probation officer, and all that tied in. And my address kicked back. And when my address kicked back, it went to Social Services. Well, I got put out. They put me out of my house. I had a house. I had a home. They put me out. They sent me a letter. I went to go walk to the mailbox to get my check, and my check was not there. It was a letter saying that my check was cut off. I had thirty days to move.

Without other means of support, Marjorie entered the HIV/AIDS system of care; however, she soon found that income generation would remain a problem in her daily life. Marjorie learned that she did not qualify for disability income because she had never been diagnosed with AIDS. In her estimation people who were eligible to receive income assistance are "more lucky than they can imagine." Perhaps not surprising, her lack of financial support translated into her resentment of "a system that don't make sense":

> I'm like, is there anywhere else I can go to apply for some help? And they like, "No because [of] this right here." We keep coming back to this. Hey, that guy has been in federal prison for six years. But you know something? He's living better than I am living. In federal prison he has cable. I don't have cable. He has radios. He has everything. He's just not free. In a way I'm not free. Because it's like I'm running into walls. Everywhere I turn, you keep those walls no matter what I do to be better. It's frustrating.

Marjorie's views of the system were largely based on her experiences with applying for and being denied monthly benefits. While cash benefits such as SSI, SSDI, and TANF can seem like luxuries to women who do not qualify for them, the realities of living on a public assistance income are not quite so appealing. For example, Ashley received $649 per month in SSI payments. She paid $300 per month for rent and approximately $150 per month for utilities. After purchasing groceries, paying for her cellular phone, and paying her monthly life insurance and car insurance premiums, Ashley's budget was at a deficit. Recognizing her relatively good health, Ashley, as did many women in this study, found employment to supplement her monthly SSI payments.[5]

Women who received less disability money than they needed sometimes turned to vocational rehabilitation (VR) services to find part-time employment. These services for disabled populations offered job and skills training that typically included programs for building skill sets required, for example, for medical transcription, legal clerical work, accounting, fiscal management, and public safety licensing. VR services also provided tuition assistance for individuals who sought education for any of the career tracks that the VR program supported. Jayla, for example, used VR services to complete a certificate in medical transcription. As we talked through our first interview together, she pointed out her framed graduation certificate for the program. At the time she completed the course, Jayla was working as a cook in a restaurant. A series of falls combined with her discomfort at being HIV-positive and working in a kitchen led Jayla to pursue a career change. She talked of how proud she felt at being a "top student" in the class. Her VR counselor had supplied Jayla with letters of recommendation and other forms of moral support for finding employment in her new field. Unfortunately Jayla's career change was not to be realized. Two months after she completed the course, Jayla had an accident and underwent several painful back surgeries that left her unable to work. Even so Jayla still viewed graduation as "one of the proudest and happiest days of [my] life."

Like Jayla, many women in this study tended to use VR services to create employment options that were less physically taxing and more flexible than construction and housekeeping. In particular VR services offered a certified nursing assistant (CNA) licensing program that was popular among the women in this study. The CNA licensing program was relatively quick, readily available, and lasted only three months on average. In addition the women, who sometimes battled fatigue and depression, saw the CNA work as "flexible." Women who found private work as a home health aide could negotiate weekly schedules with the persons they served. For example, having worked with her client for more than five years, Ashley once negotiated with her client for a three-month hiatus from her care-giving duties. Ashley frequently battled bouts of depression that coincided with painful outbreaks of genital herpes. At the onset of an outbreak that resulted in debilitating feelings of unhappiness and anxiety, Ashley felt it best to rely solely on her disability income. During this time, she visited with her daughter and bonded with her infant granddaughter. After she felt rested, Ashley was able to step back into her previous job.

Regardless of disability status, all women in good standing with Social Services qualified for the food stamps program.[6] The women had to visit their "food stamp worker" twice yearly in order to reassess and verify their need for assistance. "Need" in this context was based not only on household income and size but also on enrollment in social programs. The women were required to disclose all sources of financial support, including rent subsidies and public health care insurance, as a part of the benefits application process. Food subsidy payments ranged from $10 for single women with an income but no children to more than $300 for women with children.[7] The women who received only $10 per month were in the low-income category, but they were enrolled in other social programs that alleviated their financial burdens. Many women felt that programmatic service use should not affect their food stamp eligibility because they still struggled to make ends meet every month. Many saw the $10 assistance as an insult aimed at discouraging them from enrolling in the program altogether. Upon learning that their monthly benefits would not exceed that amount, some women in this study opted to forgo food stamps altogether.

Midway's Housing Authority also provided an invaluable source of support for many of the women in this study. While some women lived in public housing projects owned by the Housing Authority, many more sought support through the Section 8 voucher program. Section 8, as the program was popularly known, was a Housing Authority rent subsidy program for very low-income and disabled populations. To qualify the women and their families had to be in good standing with the Housing Authority, and they could not have any history of conviction for violent crime or drug-related activity. Section 8 participants were also required to keep all utilities running. If a Section 8 caseworker discovered that electricity or water services were disconnected in a Section 8 dwelling, then she or he was required to begin proceedings. Tenants had two weeks to find the money they needed to bring their bills current. If utilities were not restored within that time, the tenant faced eviction and dismissal from the Section 8 program.

Once enrolled in Section 8, adults and their families could choose an apartment or home to rent so long as the landlord accepted the Section 8 voucher. Section 8 enabled very low-income populations the opportunity to live in private residences as opposed to public housing projects. Rent was based on a sliding scale. Some women paid as little as $30 per month of their rent while others paid as much as $200 per month. The program itself was much in demand. At the time of this research, the waiting list for Section 8 enrollment was two years. New applicants were no longer being accepted.

Of all the programs that the women in this study utilized, Medicaid service use was the most widespread. Medicaid provided health insurance for the majority of them. It also provided a means for receiving fee-for-service case management. Medicaid case management differed conceptually from Ryan White case management in one important respect: Case managers billed Medicaid directly for each fifteen-minute block of time spent with a client. For every four units (one hour) of time spent with clients, Medicaid reimbursed case managers $31.50. Reimbursement was funneled through their employing organizations, which, in turn, issued paychecks minus administrative charges of anywhere from $3.00 to $7.00 per hour of service conducted.

The women in this study were well aware of the value of Medicaid health insurance with respect to case management. They also knew that case managers depended upon clients for their own income. Many women shopped around for case managers who provided them with what they felt was the best possible care. Talks of changing case managers frequently focused on the availability of a case manager and her or his willingness to "go the extra mile" for a client. In this context the extra mile could mean food pantry shopping for a client, driving a client on errands, or calling a client to see how she had been feeling. Placing such demands on case managers signified a change in the dynamics between case managers and clients.

In the past Medicaid case management functioned similar to Ryan White case management. Fee-for-service case managers provided referrals, conducted one-on-one counseling, and made phone calls on behalf of their clients. The last few years in Midway, however, saw a dramatic increase in case management agencies serving Medicaid clients. As the Ryan White dollars available for nonmedical case management dwindled and the restrictions for billing Ryan White tightened, many service agencies began solely contracting with Medicaid. In effect Medicaid case managers "flooded" the market, increasing competition for clients who had Medicaid insurance. At the time of this research there were seven Medicaid case management agencies in Midway.[8]

Some women responded to this competition skillfully. Lady E., for example, often changed case managers according to her most immediate needs and the willingness of a case manager to do what it took to win her "business." She explained, however, that the decision to change case managers was made with careful deliberation:

> Well, right now I'm in the process of changing case managers, which can always be really tricky. Because when you pulling money from people's wallets, I find basically in HIV case management that a lot of agencies don't want to take you—will not give you the services that you need because you don't have Medicaid insurance and they can't bill it to be paid. With Medicaid, you now have carte blanche. But I went a year and six months with no Medicaid. I have an allegiance to the people who hung in there with me, but at the same time if I find a agency who can service me better, I got to go with that too.

Lady E. acknowledged that "firing" a case manager could have a direct impact on her income. She also explained that personal relationships and loyalty factored into the women's decisions regarding with whom they conducted their case management business. Important also was that Lady E. received a level of service with which she felt comfortable. All of these elements shaped the dynamics between case managers and their clients, ultimately stretching the boundaries of service provision to include favors and such extras as transportation. For these reasons, the actual services that Medicaid case managers provided were highly specific to each case management relationship. Officially, however, the program focused on service coordination, the provision of referrals, and social program enrollment.

Traversing the System of Care

The programs, personnel, and procedures described here together formed an important part of the institutional context of the lives of the women in this study. The types of support, service rules, and policy regulations outlined in this chapter shaped how the women organized their time, strategized for monthly expenses, and understood what it takes to live well with HIV. They navigated this system as an integral part of their resource base. This institutional context, however, is incomplete as the life experiences of some women in this study will attest in the chapters that follow. The legal system, in-patient mental health facilities, and corporations such as rental agencies and local utility companies—all played significant roles in these women's experiences of survival with HIV disease. Moreover all of the women in this study who were navigating survival with an infectious, chronic health condition shared this institutional context. Their participation in social programs represented an observable strategy that the women utilized, albeit in different ways and to varied extents, to increase their chances for a higher quality of daily life, stability, and better health.

3. Urban Poverty Three Ways

> One-size-fits-all? See the problem with that is
> that one-size-fits-all don't fit nobody all that good.
>
> TREVA, an HIV-positive woman

As we have seen, Ryan White CARE Act programs attended to a variety of obstacles for health and survival with HIV disease. The breadth of programmatic services spanned a continuum of health-demoting conditions, including poverty, addiction, and emotional anxiety. Yet curiously absent from the system was a way to track differences in clients' access to and experiences of the continuum of care. This was perhaps, in part, because they were understood as a coherent population with fairly uniform health care needs.

Long before I began learning about the life circumstances of the individual women in this study, service providers advised me to approach service recipients in particular ways. Health Partnership employees cautioned me to "be careful" because their clients were "low income" who frequently manipulated circumstances to get extra support; that is, they lied, cheated, and stole to obtain support and donations that were not rightfully theirs. They told "sob stories" to community newcomers in the hopes of obtaining small loans, material items, and attention. I was also counseled that clients' homes were dangerous with "desperate people acting a fool." My research activities, some urged me, were best confined to Health Partnership and public places outside of the women's neighborhoods. Clients, it seemed, were a rather aggressive bunch who engaged in self-defeating strategies and had a penchant for trouble. Indeed, at times, employees gave the impression that they generally understood the conditions of violence, impoverishment, and services negotiation as individual pathology. They usually followed such advice and statements with stories implying that service providers toiled at difficult jobs for the benefit of a largely undeserving population. In this way the labels "client" and "low income" together operated as a catchall to denote an undeserving population of service recipients who failed to play by the rules and, much to the chagrin of providers, benefited from their transgressions.

Yet I found over time that most, if not all, of the service providers I met through this research cared deeply about the individual value of human lives at stake in the epidemic, as well as the lack of compassion that individuals living with HIV disease faced. I also found that many, if not most, service providers felt a personal connection and responsibility to particular clients whose lives they understood in detail, even when these clients could be considered as undeserving. Consider, for example, Greg's discussion of his "favorite" client:

> My favorite client—God rest his soul. I known him a long time. I used to see him everywhere I go. Sometimes I would see him and he'd be fine, and then I'd see him the next day and I could tell he'd been using [drugs]. He'd be acting all weird and looking sick. And he'd be hard to handle, like nobody could help him with anything. I liked him, though. He just had a problem with drugs that he couldn't kick. He got really sick, and I got word that he was in an abandoned house down the street and needed to go the hospital. I went to the house, and he was butt naked. I called an ambulance, and he wouldn't go with them. He was raising hell, yelling and talking crazy, so the ambulance wouldn't take him. So I finally got him to go with me, and I took him to the hospital myself in my car. He ended up passing away though, and it tore me up. You know, I understood him and joked around with him. A lot people didn't like him. You really see their personality and stuff like that sometimes. And I saw him everywhere. It wasn't just a job with him. He wasn't a friend, but he was part of my life.

On several occasions Greg remembered this particular client, his favorite, as a person who embodied many reasons why he chose to do this work. This man's humor and quirkiness humanized a person otherwise known only generally as part of a challenging client population. It was first through Greg's personal connection to this man that I recognized the conundrum that Health Partnership employees faced: Care providers lacked a way to reconcile "the population" created by public health policy and popular discourse with the individuals they cared about and for whom they worked often tirelessly (Bridges 2011; Foucault 1978). In other words, care providers had little choice but to ignore particular life details in this service context because they were excluded from public HIV/AIDS health care provision policy. However, in this study it was the subtle details of the women's lives that more fully explained their support service needs and the obstacles they encountered.

In this chapter I retire the one-size-fits-all category of "client" used in this setting and, instead, use categorical labels that highlight key social and material differences among the women. In so doing, I address the complexities of individual circumstance without necessarily sacrificing group-level distinctions that allow public health professionals to attend to population health. I unpack the labels "low income" and "client" while keeping in focus the general forms of inequality that all study participants encountered.

From this point I distinguish groups of women based on the differences I observed among them. These groups are organized around gradients of poverty, the women's associated daily life circumstances, and their experiences with life stressors such as mental illness, addiction, abuse, and incarceration. Poverty and life stressors have been long considered as factors confounding HIV-related health (Carovano 1991; Connors 1992; Farmer 1996; Fullilove 2006; Katz et al. 1998; McFarland et al. 2003; Remien et al. 2003; Singer 1993; Stoskopf, Richter, and Kim 2001; Tourigny 1998; Wood et al. 2002; Worth 1989). Yet until now there has been little systematic investigation of how varied combinations of material conditions and social factors articulate with HIV-related health policies and practices. Chase (2011) recently examined gradients of social capital among HIV-positive Latinas prior to the 2006 Treatment Modernization Act. Her study suggests that behaving in ways that communicate their identification with middle-class norms and values may bolster HIV-positive women's abilities to navigate the bureaucratic terrains of public health care. Successful disease management, in other words, may involve knowledge and adoption of personality traits and service use strategies that follow mainstream, middle-class logics of care and comportment. I draw from Chase to further consider the material and policy conditions of daily life that shape and complicate women's entanglements with health care providers and programs. I use the labels "stable women," "precariously situated women," and "vulnerable women" to maintain a focus on the relationships between economic conditions, social circumstances, and health care inequality.

The label "stable women" refers to the economic stability enjoyed by nine of the women in this study. The women in this group had long-term housing supported by legal entitlement to remain on the property—that is, a lease or deed in their names. Stable women also enjoyed more disposable income relative to the other women in the study. On average they earned more than $950 per month, with five women earning more than that per month. A key factor in stable women's economic stability was that they tended to have a variety of income sources, including family. Using a combination of employment, Social Security Disability Insurance, pension funds, survivor's benefits, and inheritance meant that should a problem arise with one source of income, another was available to meet short-term needs. In addition, except for Grace, whose finances were administered by a social worker specializing in support for stroke survivors, each stable woman's rental payment was no more than 30 percent of her income. These women also reported either long-term recovery (five years or more) from substance abuse or no prior history of substance abuse.

I use the categorical label "precariously situated" to illuminate the ongoing struggle half of the women faced in trying to achieve and maintain economic stability. In this group during the study period, daily life stability was often short lived, lasting only two or three months at a time. Precariously situated women rented apartments and houses in their own names. While they were legally entitled to remain on the property, this entitlement was challenged by their intermittent inability to pay rent. Most women in this group had subsidized housing, and, for some, rent subsidies capped their rental payments at 30 percent of their income. Even with rent subsidies, however, precariously situated women strategized other monthly expenses with considerably less money than their stable counterparts had. On average, women in this group earned approximately $800 per month. There was considerable range in income, however, with some women earning as little as $546 a month after garnishments and others earning more than $1,000 per month. Sources of income for members of this group were largely confined to employment and SSDI. As such, the loss of one source of income, even if partial or temporary, was devastating to the household budget. Finally most of the precariously situated women were in varying stages of substance abuse recovery. Periods of recovery for nearly all women in this group ranged from six months to five hours at the time of primary interviews.

Finally I created the category of "vulnerable women" to highlight the dire circumstances that confronted about 25 percent of the women in this study. Although *all* of the women in this study can be considered as vulnerable in relation to their low-income and health statuses, living conditions compounded the vulnerability of the women in this group. Vulnerable women were either homeless, having no legal rights to remain on any premises, or constantly cycling through eviction proceedings because they had no income to pay their rent. In fact, most of the women in this group had zero income by the end of the first research year. Two vulnerable women generated income through SSDI; however, their histories of felony conviction and active drug addiction rendered their incomes superfluous when they sought to secure an apartment lease. Unofficially women sold stolen items, participated in surveys and research studies, restored and sold items found in abandoned homes, and performed menial tasks as day laborers on construction sites. Women who did not collect Supplemental Security Insurance or SSDI payments and who did not feel well enough to work lamented their fruitless efforts to enroll in income assistance programs. Almost all vulnerable women struggled with drug addiction, incarceration, and/or mental health issues to such an extent that their economic and social viability were impeded.

While all the women in this study struggled to make ends meet each month, the types of material needs they grappled with varied according to the daily life conditions under which they strove for stability. Thus, I use the distinctions of stable, precariously situated, and vulnerable to highlight the specific pathways by which some women were better positioned than others to use HIV/AIDS care resources. To be clear these categories represent structural positions that study participants occupied in the context of federally funded HIV/AIDS care and within the specific time frame of this research. These categories, in other words, are situational and "unstable" in the sense that some women have shifted and will continue to shift between categories throughout their lives. Economic restructuring and changes in health and human services policy and in personal life circumstances have long posed both opportunities and challenges for women living in poverty. The advantage of using these categories to structure this analysis of survival is that they illuminate otherwise obscured pathways of inequality in this public health care context. Ultimately I argue that these categories shed light on specific mechanisms of inequality that pattern access to the means for HIV health and survival.

Vulnerable Women

Vulnerable women were Health Partnership's most challenging client population insofar as they lacked even the most basic resources for health and survival. They also struggled to obtain the necessary documents for service use, making it difficult for care providers to assist them in substantial ways. For this reason, in part, they struggled to meet basic survival needs such as shelter, food, and safety. The women in this group reported needs that reflected their superficial attachment to programmatic services that were outside the purview of Ryan White legislation and funding. The lack of programmatic services support was, in turn, connected to the vulnerable women's insufficient income and their poor efforts to forge and utilize strong personal support networks.

Chantelle was one vulnerable woman who faced multiple and chronic barriers for service enrollment and daily life stability. When I met Chantelle, she had been homeless for nearly thirteen years. Although only forty-five years old, the dark circles around her eyes gave her the appearance of a much older woman. Chantelle attributed this illusion to "a hard life made worse by the HIV." Chantelle's mother died when she was only eleven years old, a traumatic event that shaped her life in unimaginable ways. Her two siblings were sent to live with local relatives whom they knew well while Chantelle, the youngest, went to live with her estranged father in New Jersey. During formal interviews, she described her father as "abusive" and "a drunk." He frequently left her home alone at night, only to return intoxicated and violent. He introduced Chantelle to alcohol at age eleven and intravenous drugs at age sixteen.

At sixteen Chantelle was badly injured in a multicar accident. She sustained a broken back, fifty-four stitches in her head, and a fractured pelvis. She was eventually awarded a cash settlement for her pain and suffering, but because she was a minor, the money was entrusted to her father, who spent it at his discretion. Soon after her seventeenth birthday, Chantelle and her father moved back to Midway for reasons she did not understand. As a seventeen-year-old ninth grader, she was expelled from school for assaulting a classmate, an event that Chantelle felt marked the beginning of a long battle with the criminal justice system. Over the next five years, she was arrested an estimated fifteen times for various offenses ranging from petty theft to illicit drug possession and prostitution.

When she met and married her husband at twenty-two years old, Chantelle thought the worst of her challenges were behind her. The two lived comfortably on their sporadic incomes as day laborers, but his death in 1995 left her unable to afford the boardinghouse room they rented. At this point homeless and deeply depressed, Chantelle "basically gave up on life." Her use of illicit drugs escalated. To fund her intensifying addiction, she sold and traded sex. Later that year while "sitting in a jail cell" and serving time for charges again related to assault, Chantelle learned that she was pregnant and HIV-positive. Four months later she was released but had no money and no family willing to take her in. So began the next twelve years of Chantelle's life as a homeless and HIV-positive woman with a chemical dependency.

The first time I met Chantelle, she was looking for a service program that could help her obtain official identity documents. Chantelle's identification had been verified through her various stays at in-patient mental health facilities, prison, more than twenty stints in the local jail, and more than occasional visits to local emergency rooms; yet Social Services could not assist her beyond providing food stamps. Chantelle needed to again prove who she was to the state of North Carolina to verify her eligibility for social programs. North Carolina Department of Health and

Human Services protocol required that she obtain her New Jersey birth certificate. Her enrollment in housing subsidy programs and cash assistance services depended on it. In short, without her birth certificate, Chantelle had no institutional means for getting the help she desired. She lived with this conundrum for several months before scraping together the $15 for the document.

Once she had her ID, Chantelle needed legal assistance for settling her criminal record before Housing Authority officials could process her application. Chantelle had never fully settled formal charges brought against her for arson and check fraud. While she had served time in prison and jail for these charges, the associated fees, fines, and paperwork remained stacked against her. In the meantime, she alternated between staying with friends, checking into a recovery shelter, and sleeping outside with a group of people with whom she found safety. Frustrated and overwhelmed Chantelle lamented her predicament of being invisible and disadvantaged in the local system of care: "I can't stay in the recovery house anymore. That house is off the chain—if you ain't got one dick, you got another dick. And all of them wants me to feel it. All of them wants me to suck it. Oh, it's nasty . . . five years with this one agency and you haven't got me housing other than this? You haven't got me a job, I haven't gotten any money. What are you doing for me? Seemed like you basically helping the people that got money. I'm the one that don't have. Help me, okay?"

Over the course of this research, I came to see how conditions of homelessness and addiction posed specific barriers to Chantelle's support services eligibility. Even with proper identification, her difficult life history, HIV-positive diagnosis, and subsequent diagnoses with schizophrenia, bipolar disorder, chronic fatigue syndrome, and carpal tunnel meant Chantelle could not access services that might alleviate the desperation she felt and the poverty in which she lived. Her disqualification from SSDI exemplified these challenges in relation to AIDS care programs. As she described, "I been trying for five years now. They did decline me three times, but we appealed it this time so we're still going for it. They say I'm not eligible for disability. I can work. I can do this. I can do that. Basically, they say I'm not sick enough. I would have to have two ailments. Well, I got more than two ailments—they're just not the ailments they're looking for. Food stamps are the only thing I have."

Chantelle described a common predicament among vulnerable women. While she suffered from a variety of chronic and sometimes crippling health conditions, she did not meet the technical disability criteria for HIV disease. She had not been diagnosed with AIDS or opportunistic infections, thus she did not qualify under federal guidelines for disability status. To complicate her financial situation, Chantelle's mental health issues, often exacerbated by drug and alcohol use, left her unable to work in the formal labor market. She explained that when she was not high or drunk, she often felt too tired, achy, or depressed to meet the demands of a job. The intensity of her drug use made it altogether unlikely that she would be able to keep up with the schedule and physical demands of regular employment. Chronic fatigue and carpal tunnel syndrome further disqualified her from the informal, day-labor job market because she could not cope with the physical demands of construction work and cleaning services. As a result Chantelle remained homeless and underserved for the duration of this research study.

Jamie also faced chronic and multiple barriers to services use and stability. She survived, like all vulnerable women, without formal income and secure housing. When I met her in 2008, she had been without any income since 2000; yet she did not explain her current living conditions in relation to the loss of her most recent food service job. Like Chantelle she began her story with an explanation of her childhood. Jamie grew up in what she described as a stable family that worked hard for the few things they had. She recalled having handmade clothes and improvising meals on occasion but never feeling truly deprived. "I was optimistic," she explained, "because I had no reason not to be. My life was okay, you know." Jamie fell in love while she was young and had five children with the man she described as her "first love." However, "being young, you know, it just didn't work out. We was more in love with the idea of being in love than we really was [with] each other." When the couple separated, Jamie became an unemployed single head of household. To offset this hardship, Jamie moved her family into a local housing project. She soon "fell into the party scene" and began occasionally smoking crack with friends and neighbors. At a party one night, she met and fell in love with a man who, she later learned, was HIV-positive. Jamie learned his health status when she discovered AZT in his medicine cabinet. She promptly went for her own HIV test and discovered she too had the virus. This knowledge, she explained, intensified her addiction and led to long-term depression from which she had yet to recover: "It [the virus] made my drug use increase because—I don't know how much you know about crack, but it's like an upper. So the days that I could not function, I had my children and they got home from school and I had to function. So I would get high just to get through. And then it also helped me forget that I had this disease."

Since the escalation of her drug use habits in 2000, Jamie had been unable to abstain from smoking crack for more than a few days at a time. At first she believed that "coming to terms" with her HIV infection would curb her cravings. During our first interview, she felt as though she had accepted HIV disease as a part of her life; however, she still struggled to quit. Despite regularly attending addiction support groups and stating her desire to be sober, Jamie faced a geographical barrier to abstaining from drugs: her neighborhood was a well-known drug "hot spot." She explained how a neighbor had thwarted her latest attempt at sobriety: "I have days where I don't think about using. It just so happens up until like 6:30 this morning—because if it wasn't for them knocking on my door and me answering it—I would have three days clean. But it was someone that knew that we had gotten high—that we had bought from in the past. And it was free. That time. But I think that his sole purpose was to get me back into it."

As discussed in the introduction, dealers often gave women free tastes of crack and heroin in order to keep them as paying customers. For Jamie these offers were catastrophic to her plans for daily life stability because they complicated her ability to address other life stresses. For example, in 2004 Jamie was formally charged with child neglect, and Social Services took her children into custody. For the next few years, Jamie sold drugs and "boosted" various items to sell on the underground market.[1] Following several short-term bouts of incarceration, Jamie realized that this income-generating strategy would not help her regain custody of her children. Jamie's tragic story is rooted in poverty and a lack of access to appropriate resources to improve the whole of her circumstances, including her personal and structural vulnerabilities.

When she began trying to pull her life together in 2008, her first step was to apply for disability income so that she could have a stable environment in which to recover her health and seek custody of her children. She found, however, that over the years she had accumulated a damning arrest record, a powerful addiction to crack, and several case notes in her Social Services file that pinpointed her addiction as the primary reason she experienced poor service outcomes. These conditions affected her disability payments and her efforts to secure work. As she explained,

> I mean, my disability is like only $473 when I get it. They take some out for old fines or something. I don't think that's even the minimum, and they won't give it to me at all without a payee. I mean, these are people who need these things for their lives. Like, for me, it's hard to get a job because I have a record that includes theft. Even though I dealt with it, it's still on my record, so when they pull it up, all they can see is what I used to be. But that's not who I am trying to be now.

Jamie felt she was ready to move beyond the self-defeating survival strategies she had employed in the past. She said she was willing to adhere to programmatic service rules as a means of demonstrating her commitment to changing her life. This long-term commitment, however, was difficult to maintain in the face of short-term needs. For example, in order to receive ssdi, Jamie was legally required to have a payee unrelated to her by blood or marriage. While she looked for an appropriate payee whom she could trust, Jamie was unable to receive her check. She therefore struggled to afford food, medications, and household utilities. Further complicating these struggles was the fact that she had no legal rights to her house. Because she lived in her partner's home, she was thus technically homeless.

For vulnerable women such as Jamie and Chantelle who found themselves with few options for income and secure housing, food stamps were a vital resource. Indeed, they sometimes meant the difference between sleeping outside and the relative comfort of sleeping on a friend's couch. Food stamps could be traded for a number of necessities, including money, drugs, and physical protection; however, like many valuable resources, they were not easy to obtain. And for women who had few formally documented financial burdens to prove their need, they were nearly impossible to get. The problem, according to vulnerable women, was that some Social Services case workers refused to distribute food stamps unless the applicant had a lease or utility bills in their names. Many women were denied food stamps or given only the minimum allotment of $10 per month because of this technicality.

Given this intense lack of basic necessities, Midway's vulnerable women relied upon the support of personal social networks. Vulnerable women frequently maintained long-established social networks and used them often, even though they were initially forged and maintained through illicit drug use. These networks nonetheless functioned as a safety net for women who had few other options for getting help.

Tasha was one woman whose friends proved a valuable network of support during an otherwise stressful life. When we first sat down together for a formal discussion and interview, just days before Tasha had completed a prison sentence for arson charges. Her personal life story was shaped in her youth by years of sexual violence and abuse by her older brother. She also lived with the haunting memory of being raped by a White stranger. Fearful of stigma and shame, Tasha never shared with her family the realities of the sexual violence she suffered. She instead "kept it secret because I knew they [her family] would blame me." Tasha linked the violence and the emotional turmoil they engendered to her subsequent battles with chemical dependency. As she explained, "I didn't just wake up and say, 'Hey, I want to smoke crack.' Raped when I was sixteen, and then I started smoking crack. Out there tricking, selling on that corner, selling my body. And then I got raped again when I was, like, thirty-nine, right on the street. It was a White guy too. So yeah, so you know. I didn't call the police because I felt like, 'Hey, I'm out there selling to make some money.' I figured I was in the wrong. What the hell."

Tasha plainly identified sexual assault as a primary reason for her subsequent battles with addiction. Further, the emotional abuse and neglect she suffered shaped her fateful decision to set her family's home on fire. Her family members escaped physically unharmed, but they pressed charges and had her arrested. Her parole conditions prohibited any contact with her family. She therefore had nowhere else to turn after her release but to those friends with whom she had previously used illicit drugs.

Tasha's friends invited her to stay with them while she reinstated her disability payments and completed the probationary period following her incarceration; however, the conditions under which she lived were less than desirable. Her roommate frequently made unwanted sexual advances. When Tasha refused his advances, he retaliated by locking her out of the house and not allowing her to use the bathroom indoors. As she explained the situation, "Half the time he was making me piss outside in the trash can—it was crazy. And then, you know, I was kicking out—because wherever I go, of course you know I'm going to pay my way. I ain't sleeping with nobody just because I need a favor. Yeah, you letting me stay, but I will pay you something. It got to be where I had no choice but to leave."

Tasha did eventually leave that situation. She considered herself lucky because she had another "party friend" who offered his support. He was also HIV-positive and so shared Tasha's concern for privacy. In addition, this friend did not coerce Tasha to perform sexual favors in lieu of financial contributions to the household. Together they tried to abstain from using drugs and alcohol, but they found sobriety difficult to achieve. After a few months, Tasha's friend was gravely ill, and she felt it was time to leave again. Tasha's disability payments had been reinstated by this time. She was receiving close to $900 per month in disability payments, but she was still unable to secure an apartment of her own. Property managers were unwilling to rent to someone convicted of arson. She soon moved in with another friend until the landlord evicted them both so that he could move to Midway and live in the property himself. Tasha then began alternating between staying at the local shelter and renting hotel rooms. When I returned to Midway in 2009, Tasha was still cycling between hotels and homeless shelters.

As Tasha's story suggests, homelessness leaves women dependent on personal social networks for shelter and basic survival needs. The demands placed on women in these arrangements were emotionally taxing. They often found themselves in coercive or abusive living arrangements. The emotional toll imparted through challenging conditions of financial want and physical vulnerability should not be underestimated as a life detail relevant to health. Indeed, the vulnerable women in this study emphasized the misery they felt in connection to their living conditions and the burdens they shouldered simply to maintain their functioning social networks.

Rosalind, for example, often cried during our discussions and interviews. She lamented that she lived "the life of a hermit" because she feared disclosure of her HIV-positive status. She explained during our first interview that she lived with her mother and son in a neighborhood controlled by one of the local gangs. Her fear of violent crime exacerbated the stress she often felt in relation to her poverty and life with HIV disease. Having food stamps as her only form of income, Rosalind relied on neighbors, friends, and family for financial assistance. Rosalind additionally suffered with spinal arthritis. Many mornings she needed assistance to get out of bed. Her pain was constant and exhausting. Neither the arthritis nor her HIV status, though, qualified her for disability income. As a former medical records clerk at a local hospital, she knew too well how employees sometimes discussed the health records and medical charts they tracked and filed. Rosalind thus used an alias at the physician's office and avoided any discussions of health with those to whom she turned for support, including her mother and son. She described her fear of being "found out" as emerging from self-preservation: "To avoid it [social contact] means not putting yourself in the position to meet that person who needs to know. People in the world are very ignorant. They do not know that there is life after the virus. I just don't know that it's my job to teach people that at my expense. . . . That expense is feeling like you're 'less than,' being treated like you're less than because you got it. Being cut off." Rosalind's decision to keep her HIV diagnosis private thus protected her from social abandonment. It both shielded her from negative reactions and judgment and helped to ensure that members of her personal social network would continue offering the material support she needed.

Over time Rosalind grew weary of keeping secrets. She avoided going to Health Partnership during its peak hours lest she see an acquaintance who might gossip. She began calling program employees from the parking lot and asking who was inside before entering. While at the organization, she seemed agitated and constantly watched the front door, frequently describing her fears of seeing fellow Health Partnership clients in public. Sick with paranoia and "tired of the hustle," Rosalind decided to disclose her status to her brother. His initial response was supportive and kind. However, during an argument a few months later, Rosalind's brother told her that he was glad that she was dying of HIV. Rosalind felt betrayed, distraught, and emotionally wounded by his insensitive remarks. This devastating blow led Rosalind to voluntarily commit herself to an in-patient psychiatric facility for several weeks. Rosalind, like other vulnerable women, continued to struggle to maintain her social network, a task unequivocally important for women lacking access to basic necessities and support service programs.

Precariously Situated Women

Precariously situated women, although housed and enrolled in income support programs, coped with persistent fluctuations in monthly resources. The relatively high proportions of income they spent on monthly rental payments, coupled with fewer actual sources of support, meant that women in this group frequently carried a portion of each month's bills over to the next month. This strategy, although viable in the short term, usually led to periodic eviction and disconnection of their utilities. Thus their needs and living conditions changed frequently and suddenly. Women in this group often responded to questions about their financial circumstances that they were "doing fine at the moment" or were "not too good this week." Their responses almost always included a reference to the present as an indication that their situations could change or had recently changed. Perhaps for this reason, precariously situated women identified a broad range of needs and struggles.

Women in this group qualified for a variety of social programs outside the system of HIV care, but they often had trouble coordinating the technical demands of service eligibility rules and procedures for the various programs that might meet their needs. Enrollment and continuing eligibility protocols can be daunting tasks for the precariously stable because they require keeping meticulous records and maintaining sometimes-complicated appointment schedules. Facing the daily burdens of affording food, shelter, and other basic provisions on a small income can make a seemingly simple task such as completing paperwork feel as if it is one more obstacle to overcome.

Tanya, for example, was a twenty-six-year-old mother of seven for whom the tasks of daily life and household maintenance were overwhelming. When we first met, she was four months pregnant with twins and had full custody of four of her five other children. She complained of debilitating fatigue and how difficult it made her daily life. Laundry, meal preparation, child discipline, physician appointments, informal income generation, and Parent-Teacher Association activities filled Tanya's daily schedule from morning until night. To intensify an already overwhelming schedule, Tanya was anxious about her babies' potential health problems. She felt that she had been lucky to give birth to five HIV-negative children and feared that she would not be as fortunate with this pregnancy. Even so as a former ward of the state, Tanya felt that a large family was a "dream come true, even if it's not always easy."

Tanya lived in what she described as "almost total chaos." The family lived in a three-bedroom apartment in a housing project on the outskirts of town. Tanya's husband, who was also HIV-positive, suffered from depression and occasional bouts of frustration and anger. His emotional instability made it difficult for him to maintain regular employment. Tanya struggled under these conditions to satisfy her family's needs. As she described their financial situation in January 2008, "It's tight sometimes. The kids need stuff. I don't have a light bill or any of that stuff though. I don't have any rent. I got HUD [U.S. Department of Housing and Urban Development] housing so they pay my rent. I have zero income officially. I do that tutoring on the side, but I don't have to pay any taxes on it so it shows up as zero income. That's how I wash clothes, get detergent, buy those extra things, you know. So it's, like, $80 or $100 a month that I bring in. I make money."

Tanya was technically able to make ends meet through a public housing program, informal income generation, WIC vouchers, and the additional $425 she received every month in food stamps. She still needed more income support for "extras" such as clothing, telephone service, personal care items, and educational toys for her youngest children. Temporary Assistance for Needy Families was one option that Tanya had exhausted and now sorely missed. (She had already met her lifetime eligibility limit of five years.) Though her status as a pregnant former ward of the state with four small children already positioned her to receive "extra" Social Services support, Tanya could not figure out how to make her claim for that support. As she described,

> They make it really hard for you to get that. You got to have birth cer-
> tificates, IDs. You got to have all that for each child and for yourself. I
> have it for my kids, but I don't have a birth certificate for me. It's in
> New Jersey somewhere. I don't have any idea how to get a hold of that
> and prove to them that I'm me requesting it. The lady told me that I
> had to have a birth certificate before they could process my applica-
> tion. I'm like, are you kidding? I was a ward of the state. I been getting
> welfare, Medicaid, and food stamps in this state since I was ten years
> old. I just don't have the time to run around everywhere for this.

Many women like Tanya who lived in unstable conditions did without some of the support to which they were technically entitled because they did not want the added burden of adhering to programmatic service rules and regulations. Doing without a programmatic service in this scenario was a strategy for avoiding time-consuming and sometimes emotionally draining enrollment and eligibility maintenance procedures.

Given the women's decisions to forgo the full range of programmatic services, many precariously situated women lived in challenging, if not dangerous, housing conditions. Although technically "housed" because they were loosely protected by rental contracts, their homes lacked many of the features and basic household necessities associated with quality housing such as refrigerators, working stoves and ovens, furniture, and, in a couple of cases, kitchen utensils. Women made do the best way they could devise. Makeshift furniture, plastic utensils from local fast food restaurants, and large appliances covered with tattered sheets and pic-ture frames were telltale signs of the women's struggles to accumulate the material convenience items that many Americans take for granted in their homes.

Over the course of the research, Tanya's life was further complicated by material want. She improvised as best she could when she, her hus-band, and her (then) six children were evicted from public housing in

June 2008 because they could not afford to keep their utilities running. Social Services did assist the family with a deposit and the first month's rent for a new, unsubsidized apartment; however, Tanya's income as a part-time cleaning woman meant that they could afford little. After hasty preparation, the family moved into an apartment that did not have a refrigerator or a stove. Within one week of moving, Tanya found closer to full-time employment as a cashier at a fast food restaurant. She managed to scrape together the money for a stove, but five months later, she still did not have a refrigerator.

The wages Tanya earned as a cashier at the restaurant paid only her rent and utilities. Earning $6.75 per hour, or roughly $930 per month, she had no choice but to supplement her income with food stamps, clothing donations, and food pantries. The added burden of having to live without a refrigerator was, by this point, "so ridiculous that [she] just can't even care." Tanya kept perishable food in a cooler, bought small portions, and returned to the store frequently throughout the week. In the end having no refrigerator cost Tanya additional money for transportation to the grocery store. She also frequently lost food that might otherwise have been eaten as leftovers or stored in the freezer for later use. As she described her abilities to cope with recent misfortune, "I can jump in there and work. I'll probably keep us all afloat, but as far as getting us back to the shore—I swim like a rock—better hope I can just float here."

Tanya described her recent foray into food service industry employment in terms of "jumping in" the water. The shore, in her estimation, represents a time when she, her husband, and her children enjoyed greater stability afforded by social programs such as public housing and TANF. After being disqualified from those services, her only choice was to work, however low the wages and unstable the hours. This strategy—indeed, the one that social program guidelines preferred—seemed more like sinking than swimming to her. Tanya felt her only recourse was to hope that she could get by until she found a new apartment or a better job. In general, however, precariously situated women did not experience much luck in terms of finding new or improved housing that fit their budgets. While many women frequently moved into new apartments, their moves could often be considered as either lateral or, in some ways, regressive.

Lady E. was one woman who had endured a series of lateral housing moves over the course of this research project. At the time of our first interview, she was living in a modest rental house she could not technically afford. Lady E. earned zero income, but with the help of Social Services, Health Partnership, and state-funded addiction recovery and mental health programs, she managed to pay her monthly rent and utilities. Health Partnership programs also covered her medical expenses, food, and transportation. For three months Lady E. relearned "how to live everyday life without drugs" with few financial worries. During this time she focused on developing her hobbies (crocheting and beading) and on recovering her health. She had been diagnosed with AIDS long ago, but her CD4 cell and viral load counts had steadily improved since her sobriety. Lady E. also suffered from a serious heart condition and had recently undergone a ninth angioplasty and endured two heart attacks. Given her health problems, Lady E. felt the housing assistance she received was "a godsend."

After three months, however, the addiction recovery program expected Lady E. to become self-sufficient; that is, she would need to pay her own rent and utilities in addition to finding more permanent solutions to food insecurity, transportation needs, and medication copays. Lady E. feared going back to a recovery house or a homeless shelter where "people aren't serious about their sobriety." She thus wasted no time applying for disability insurance, food stamps, and Medicaid. Given her health history and AIDS diagnosis, she qualified for disability insurance with relatively little hassle. Yet Lady E. soon found that $650 per month in disability payments and $90 per month in food stamps was not conducive to self-sufficiency. She then opted to move into a boardinghouse.

Lady E. regretted having to leave the rental house, as it was spacious, clean, and private, if too expensive. In her estimation, moving to the boardinghouse was simultaneously a "step forwards and a step backwards." Her new room was affordable; at just $375 per month, she could consistently pay her rent. She took a big step toward independent living and daily life stability. Her new room was also very small, however, so she had to give away some personal belongings. Her room, not much bigger than a ten-by-ten-foot storage locker, held less than half of what Lady E. had accumulated over forty-nine years. She managed to fit a twin bed, a dresser, a bookshelf, a nightstand, a desk, a microwave, and numerous baskets of stuffed animals, beads, yarn, and trinkets in the small space. Her clothes hung from exposed pipes in the ceiling, making the space seem disheveled and haphazard despite her best efforts. When I first helped her move in, Lady E. explained that the room was "small, but it's mine, you know? I can pay for this. This is mine, and it's my doing." She was also optimistic that fellow renters did not seem to "live the party life."

Unfortunately Lady E.'s optimism turned to despair when her food began to disappear from the communal kitchen. She also developed a persistent wet cough that exacerbated an already troublesome case of asthma. She asked the landlord numerous times about the possibility of mold in her room. She was fairly certain that her personal space had been once used as a toolshed. It had the only private entrance off the back of the house, and she suspected that the wood paneling in her room concealed mold. After two months of getting the run around from her lessor, one three-day hospitalization, and the addition of a portable oxygen tank to her already burdensome health care regimen, Lady E. called the city's housing inspection services. An inspector promptly identified the issue and labeled the room as "unfit for human occupation."

Lady E.'s next housing situation proved no more conducive to stability than either of the other two although for very different reasons. Again she moved into a boardinghouse. Her room was bigger and included a dormitory-size refrigerator. She paid slightly more for this room, at $395 per month, but she felt it was worthwhile because the house was near a college campus. She planned to sell her beadwork to students as means of making up the difference in rent. Lady E.'s first month in this new house seemed to go smoothly. She met and liked a couple of her neighbors. The house itself was near the main bus lines, and her room was clear of pests and mold. At this time Lady E. began feeling confident that she was going to achieve the financial stability and daily life normalcy she longed for. She began attending fewer substance abuse meetings, cutting attendance from three times a week to once a week. She also began socializing on a local "party chat line," where she met other single people who were "lonely and looking to just have a good laugh." She prided herself on getting her monthly disability check and "not needing to spend it on drugs." Instead, she spent her time teaching children how to make jewelry at a local after-school recreation center. She also tutored young children in a chapter of the Boys & Girls Club. When I exited the field in November 2008, Lady E. had just received notice that she had been verified for the Section 8 program. She needed only to clear up outstanding debts to the power company. In short, Lady E. was "making it."

By the following January, Lady E.'s stability had wavered. She was hospitalized six times between January and March with her heart condition. During this time, her daughter moved out of town, leaving her with few options for social activities and personal support. Since she had stopped intensively attending substance abuse support group meetings, she felt returning to her old support group schedule would be tantamount to defeat. She instead turned to her fellow boardinghouse tenants, some of whom used drugs. She soon began smoking crack with them, occasionally at first. Eventually her use escalated into a two-week crack binge, during which she spent her disability back pay, lost her Section 8 eligibility, was evicted from her room, and lost the city grant money she received for her work with local children's groups. As she described, "I smoked a ball a day or better. I went through the first two thousand dollars in, like, a week and a half. Okay, I was smoking day and night. I actually in twenty-seven years of addiction had the opportunity to smoke, not just until the money ran out—I still had money—I was able to smoke until I didn't want it. That's why I passed on any more. I really just didn't want it."

When Lady E. described her binge to me in June 2009, she was three weeks sober. Her previous experience and success with substance abuse programs translated into expedited enrollment in a local recovery house. Lady E. was optimistic about addiction recovery because she had the support of several organizations, including Health Partnership. Recovering her health, however, was a different challenge. Lady E.'s heart condition continued to worsen, despite her best efforts at sobriety, treatment adherence, and healthy eating. I received an email in December of that year letting me know that Lady E. had died. The poignancy of her observations during our interview from that summer remains emblazoned in my mind: "The party's over. Take my dancing shoes off."

Even amid the gravity of Lady E.'s housing struggle, it should be noted that precariously situated women described how they "loved" where they lived as often as they lamented their housing options. They almost always compared this love to their past experiences of homelessness or of living with relatives who either feared HIV infection or who did not know about HIV infection. Indeed, many precariously situated women have dealt with the disappointments and surprises that accompany disclosing their health status to loved ones. Thus having an apartment or house of one's own afforded some women a safe space to return when loved ones rejected them after learning their HIV-positive status. In other cases moving into and maintaining one's own apartment enabled the women to take another step toward stability and living well with HIV disease. Even if it did not necessarily mean that the women enjoyed financial stability, as Lady E. said, having their own apartments afforded them a sense of "just having your life somewhat together and, you know, being, like, you can take care of yourself."

In addition to housing challenges, precariously situated women frequently lamented the small stipends they received as income assistance. For all SSI and SSDI recipients, the amount of income assistance received is based on household size and the history of Social Security taxes and payroll taxes paid. Although many precariously situated women had formal work histories, they had always been considered under Social Service's guidelines as categorically low income; that is, the women in this group had not paid enough in Social Security taxes to receive much more than the minimum monthly allotment of income assistance. Most precariously situated women in this study also had only themselves to report as household members and, as a result, received a monthly insurance stipend of only about $623. However, whether this income was sufficient to meet their needs was shaped by a variety of life factors and circumstances often beyond the consideration of individual federal program employees or federal poverty guidelines.

For example, the women's legal histories and household composition affected their eligibility claims for in-kind resources and, in turn, the efficacy of monthly disability payments. Treva was one woman who found that her SSDI payments were not enough to meet all of her basic needs, let alone the needs of her disabled partner. Treva migrated from

New Jersey to Midway in 2000. She was tired of New Jersey and wanted to leave her past behind. She was tested and diagnosed as HIV-positive when she gave birth to her second-born son in 1991. At first Treva "kept it together for the sake of that little one [her son]." She refused treatment and follow-up testing for her baby because she "didn't feel sick and so couldn't believe it." She and her younger son moved to be near her elder child, who had recently been transferred to work in the area. Upon arrival, however, Treva found her lack of a high school diploma was a liability in Midway's overcrowded labor market. She was unable to find work and felt it unfair for her to ask her son for financial support. Treva quickly applied for benefits from Social Services, which initially rejected her from enrollment. It seemed a clerical error confused her with a woman of the same name who owed the state rental housing back pay. During this time Treva's young son became gravely ill. He received state-sponsored health insurance and was diagnosed and treated for AIDS-related complications. He died late in 2001, a tragedy for which Treva blamed herself. "I still feel guilty about that," she explained, "I feel that it's my fault he died. I really do."

When Treva's benefits were finally approved in 2005, they were proportioned to her life circumstances as a legally single woman with no children at home, but she consistently ran out of food and had trouble paying her bills. As she explained the perpetual financial predicament she faced, it became clear that federal guidelines do not take into account all the factors complicating women's lives and needs. Principal for Treva was her history of drug addiction and a felony conviction for which she had served time but continued to "pay for" in the form of being disqualified from particular programs. She explained, "I was on methadone. I wrote a prescription for methadone and got caught. I did a hundred twenty-three days. And that disqualified me because it was considered a felony. So now I can't get no food stamps. That really stresses me out real bad. I paid for it. You know, I'm on probation, and I'm still paying. I called Legal Aid, and they were supposed to send me some paperwork that might help, but I don't know what's up."

Treva's felony conviction for prescription fraud disqualified her from participation in the state's food stamp program. Her grocery budget now necessarily cut into a monthly income that was already stretched thin by rent and utilities payments. On just $623 per month, she paid $450 per month in rent, roughly $80 per month for utilities, $35 per month for a local telephone, and up to $12 per month for medication copayments. These expenses left Treva with about $50 per month for groceries and incidentals such as cleaning supplies and personal care items. She punctuated our discussion about her economic struggles with the realization that "this month I have been to four pantries, and I still don't have food in my refrigerator. They [the state] just set you up to fail—or steal—when they cut you off like that. Their solution is for me to go to food pantries all week long. I don't think that's helping. They just keep punishment up because of my past."

Unfortunately a few weeks after our conversation, Treva dropped out of support services at Health Partnership. She remained out of contact with program employees and me for the duration of this research. Dropping out or "laying low" was a common, though usually temporary, occurrence among women who felt that programmatic services could not address their issues in any significant way. Frustration and emotional fatigue led them to the idea that program participation was not worth the effort it took to maintain enrollment.

As described earlier, the women who were considered as precariously situated were often on the brink either of economic collapse or of thriving relatively comfortably. As explained in relation to vulnerable women, personal social support networks could mediate housing status, material lack, insufficient income, and the eligibility demands of programmatic services. Yet most precariously situated women were also in various stages of substance abuse recovery and/or had variously revealed to family and friends their health concerns. The emotional and social upheavals associated with disclosure and addiction recovery meant that members of this group tended to have few, if any, operative social network members. For women in this group, having few supportive individuals to turn to often led to coercive and/or abusive relationships. In contexts of social and economic upheaval, personal support networks presented barriers to living well while simultaneously facilitating material comfort or advantage. Lisa's living conditions and small support network illuminate this predicament.

Lisa was one of the few women in this research who lived in what she described as a "comfortable home in a safe neighborhood." As with all women described as precariously situated, she utilized several social programs, including SSDI, food stamps, Medicaid, food pantries, and emergency assistance programs. According to Lisa, however, her greatest resource was her personal network, which in some ways amplified the benefits of receiving programmatic services. At the same time, however, Lisa was vulnerable to the demands of the few network members who supported her efforts to live well.

Although she came from a self-identified working-class background, she had never felt the same desire her siblings had for "that picket fence life." I met two of Lisa's siblings, financially successful women who loved Lisa and looked after her from a respectful distance. Yet despite their enduring support and my gentle prodding, Lisa rarely discussed her childhood or natal family other than to celebrate memories of her mother and father whom she loved dearly and remembered kindly.

Her story of HIV survival began when her baby sister died of AIDS-related complications in 1995. At that time Lisa was unaware of her own status because she was "still doing drugs and didn't care to know." She remembered watching her sister "wear diapers and waste away in a wheelchair." These traumatic memories shaped Lisa's decision not to be tested, despite that she had shared needles and had had unprotected sex with individuals she suspected were HIV-positive. A few years later when Lisa decided to "get clean," she recognized the symptoms: fatigue, night sweats, and general achiness. An emergency room visit confirmed her suspicion. Lisa immediately began antiretroviral therapy.

After diagnosis Lisa spent two years being homeless, "hustling," and falling in love with her long-term partner, Layla. The two slept under bridges and panhandled until Lisa grew weary of living outdoors. She checked into a local rehabilitation facility, only to find that it had given her the last bed. Her partner, suffering from untreated schizophrenia, was left on her own. Lisa quickly decided that she "could handle the world better than her [partner]" and coordinated her own checkout with Layla's admission. When Lisa's partner checked herself out of the shelter after three days, Lisa, angry with this decision, physically beat Layla and then spent several days "getting drunk and showing [her] ass." Lisa finally called one of her sisters to come get her when she realized how out of control she had been.

Lisa's sister promptly took her to the hospital, and Lisa learned "just how bad it [the HIV] had got." Years of crack use, alcohol abuse, and sleeping outdoors had taken its toll on her health. She felt herself near death, a premonition confirmed by her low CD4 cell count and high viral load. Her physician explained that the disease had progressed to AIDS. It was then that Lisa decided to "take control and be a survivor of this disease." Lisa enrolled in several AIDS-related social programs, including an HIV support group, medical care, and case management. She also retained free legal help for applying for disability insurance benefits. Her diagnosis with AIDS and associated opportunistic infections qualified her for federal income assistance. She reunited with Layla during her stay at a state-funded transitional housing unit. Layla had enrolled in mental health care programs, had applied for mental health–related disability benefits, and had quickly applied for and received a Section 8 housing voucher. The pair, now both hooked into state programs and services, found a rental house in a middle-class neighborhood outside the downtown area.

It was at this point that I met Lisa. At the time she felt indebted to Layla because, despite the abuse, Layla chose to share her resources with Lisa and her two teenage daughters. Lisa often spoke of how much she cared for her partner. She recounted how they met, drifted apart, and came back together as proof that they were destined to share their lives. However, her partner's mental health issues and their shared addiction to illicit drugs sometimes complicated Lisa's feelings of love and admiration. The practical dimensions of maintaining a household under conditions of poverty, mental instability, and addiction were overwhelming at best. Yet even should the worst of times arrive, Lisa felt that she could not just simply leave her partner. She emphasized that without her partner's disability income, she would still be homeless and "running the streets." She also could not afford to care for her daughters and remain in their three-bedroom rental house. Despite her sometimes-rocky relationship with her partner, Lisa explained:

I can't thank her enough. It's just what we have to do because that little $637 is not enough. I would have to live in a rooming house. The rent is $200 to $300 in the ghetto. Then you got to pay a light bill, and how am I going to take my daughters somewhere in the ghetto? Oh, a crack house—sure, no problem. Then you got a water bill, a light bill, the sewer, or whatever. And I just thank God for her because I wouldn't be able to do it. I would have to live in a rooming house. I had my experiences in a rooming house. And my babies were still with me, and my daughters would come home from school in that environment. It's not fair to them.

Lisa recognized that she could not afford to raise her daughters in a safe environment by herself. This realization guided her decision to use drugs, a strategy with obvious implications for her recovery goals. For example, one afternoon Lisa's daughters answered the door upon my arrival at their home. They asked to talk to me alone outside because they were worried about their mom, and they did not want Layla to hear them. The girls explained that Lisa had been in recovery. She had been smoking cigarettes and drinking beer, but she had not smoked crack in close to three weeks. Layla, however, had begun trying to coerce Lisa into smoking. She threatened to leave and withhold money from Lisa and the girls if Lisa did not smoke with her. Lisa came outside and lamented the precarious position in which she found herself; however, she noted that "it could be worse if we were homeless. Then what would we do?"

In Lisa's case having to cope with her sometimes-difficult relationship was put into sharp focus when in 2009 she inherited close to $35,000 from her mother. After garnishments Lisa had a little less than half of the money left. She knew, however, that $17,000 would not make a difference in her life for long but believed that it could potentially disqualify her from receiving SSDI payments. She entrusted the money to her sister and periodically used it for cruise vacations with her daughters and for small home improvements such as carpet and upholstery cleaning. Lisa viewed using the inheritance money to pay rent or utilities or simply to build a nest egg as potentially damaging to her long-term stability because, per SSDI eligibility rules, the money would be an asset factored into her monthly income payments. Lisa also feared that if Social Security found out about the money, they would ask her to pay back what she had collected in disability payments. Lisa felt that the money was most useful in smaller increments over the long-term future. Had she used the money to move into an apartment or house of her own, she would eventually face, once again, being unable to afford monthly bills. Lisa instead remained with Layla and focused her efforts on modestly improving their existing living conditions. Thus as did other precariously situated women, Lisa stayed put in the position of being one step away from thriving and one step away from "eating it."

This precariousness was especially evident when I reconnected with Lisa in May 2012. Layla had decided approximately a year earlier that she no longer wanted to be in a same-sex relationship. She accused Lisa of manipulating her mental and emotional instability as a means of obtaining money and housing. Layla moved out of their house, so Lisa had no choice but to leave too. Lisa next moved into an apartment that she described as "a real shit-hole that was lousy with cockroaches. I got in there because I didn't want to be homeless on the street. And it was a one-bedroom apartment with a living room and kitchen. We had to have gas heat and I couldn't afford the gas heat because they wanted a $300 deposit and my check is only $698. Well, now my check is $698. At the time it was a little cheaper than that. So the rent was only $400, so it was affordable. I used electric heaters, and then sometimes I had air-conditioned windows."

During this time Lisa's drinking and anxiety escalated. She also frequently missed medication doses and physician appointments. "I was having panic attacks every day," she said. "I felt like somebody was coming after me. I couldn't be alone so I would have to sit with somebody all day. And the person I would go sit with was drinking so then I was drinking." Amid all of this, Lisa's son had lost his job and moved in with her. Then four people were living in the roach-infested one-bedroom apartment.

Over that winter Lisa's asthma worsened, and she chose to leave the apartment. One big problem, however, was that Lisa could not afford to hire a moving crew or rent a truck. She moved only what she and her children could carry on the bus.

I mean, I had food for ya—I had a deep freezer full of food, turkeys in it and everything. I lost food. I mean, nothing is really hard to replace because I'm still alive. Material things like that, I don't know. I told my children, "Get what you need," because they had their stuff in there too. They had their shoes, you know. I took my TVs. I left behind two beds, a loveseat and couch, an entertainment stand, a lot of clothes, towels, washcloths, food, a grill, a lot of my pots and pans, silverware, glasses, air conditioners, heaters—sure did.

Thus at the time of our last interview in 2012, Lisa was living in a near-empty apartment that cost more than 70 percent of her monthly income. She paid $500 per month in rent but received only $698 per month in SSDI payments. Perhaps needless to say, she, like other precariously situated women, continued to struggle intermittently with sobriety, social distress, and material want.

Stable Women

Stable women's material conditions were often less stressful than those of their precariously situated and vulnerable counterparts. Stable women tended more frequently to struggle with satisfying material needs that the various support services viewed as being of secondary importance in relation to housing, hunger, and health insurance. Some stable women met their primary needs, such as housing and income, long ago by enrolling in social programs. Other stable women addressed their primary needs with income generated through employment, pensions, and inheritance. In most cases they satisfied primary needs through a combination of programmatic services and employment; however, the secondary needs that stable women identified are also significant for experiences of health. I thus do not want to suggest that stable women's material needs are any less urgent than what was reported by vulnerable and precariously situated women; rather, I suggest that stable women's material needs represent another interlocking set of circumstances along a continuum of HIV health needs and survival experiences.

Stable women, as noted, generated income through various resources including spousal support, SSI, SSDI, pensions, part-time or full-time work, and inheritance. Using a combination of income assistance programs and economic resources meant that they had greater incomes than precariously situated women and vulnerable women. On average they enjoyed about 30 percent more money each month than their precariously positioned counterparts. This cushion translated into feelings of financial viability and optimism, despite the women's status as "low income." DeeDee, for example, understood herself as financially viable despite being categorically low income. When I met her, she was providing live-in care for her elderly mother, who was recovering from hip replacement surgery. While sharing the costs of living with her mother, DeeDee received a $1,167 monthly pension for her previous career in the U.S. military and, at the time of our first interview, earned approximately $700 per month for part-time clerical work she found through a local temporary employment agency. DeeDee also utilized Health Partnership's food pantry on a regular basis. Supplementing her groceries enabled her to save money for a future home and a car of her own. She additionally searched for full-time employment, carefully seeking career work paying more than the minimum wage. As a high school graduate with some college experience and a former military career, DeeDee expected to earn no less than $10 an hour. Though she was unable to find secure work during the study period, she managed to save close to $500 each month. She generated enough income that she neither qualified for nor wanted disability insurance payments. She explained, "I pay my own way. I just don't need all the support that some other women might need. I might come down here and get my little foods, but I'd be okay without it too. I just couldn't save as much."

Grace, on the contrary, needed and utilized multiple social programs that together kept her financially stable and relatively comfortable. Grace was a former public school teacher who could no longer work. During a two-week whirlwind in 2004, Grace suffered from a serious stroke that left her partially paralyzed with mild mental impairment. She also learned at that time that she was HIV-positive and, by implication, discovered her husband's infidelity. To say that Grace was devastated by this overwhelming news is an understatement. She cried frequently throughout formal interviews but insisted that others should know her story because it is ultimately one of triumph and strength.

When she was initially released from the hospital, Grace's case manager enrolled her in the ssi program, food stamps, and two stroke survivor support groups. Grace's teaching career also provided her with a small pension for her service. Although she was unsure exactly how much she collected each month from ssi and her pension, she knew she had the basic resources that she needed to make ends meet every month. Grace's case manager additionally arranged for her to have a payee, a social worker who was employed by a local hospital, to ensure her bills were paid each month. She qualified for the hospital payee program specifically because of her stroke and the brain injury from which she suffered as a result. Her payee, "Mr. Eric," paid $630 per month in rent and approximately $200 per month for cable, telephone services, and electricity. Mr. Eric reserved $100 per month for Grace to spend as she felt necessary. Grace used this money to supplement the $179 per month she received in food stamps and to purchase cleaning products and personal care items. She often requested more spending money, but Mr. Eric explained to her that her budget was already stretched too thin. In fact, Mr. Eric sometimes requested emergency assistance from hospital programs and Social Services on Grace's behalf. No matter what her financial situation, Mr. Eric made sure that she had at least that little bit of cash on hand. Grace knew that she was more financially viable than many women living on public assistance, but nonetheless she lamented her frequent lack of disposable income for secondary needs:

> I'm paying $630 a month in rent. And then my light bill and my phone, and my cable. I have a life insurance policy. Sometimes the light bill is being paid for by Mr. Eric—not even my money. And he pays my cable when I can't too. And I get my food stamps. So then he don't have nothing to give for me to buy my makeup or buy my shower gel or stuff that women needs, cosmetics and stuff. I don't have money for that. It's just hard because those are the things that make you feel pretty, like when you see other people when you go out. I used to be a schoolteacher, and I could buy the things I needed. Now I can't even wear makeup like a normal woman does.

Although Grace had clear access to shelter and food, she still had material wants and needs. In particular, Grace longed for material items such as the cosmetics and shower gels that she felt were conducive to her mental and social health. And in 2009 Grace implemented a strategy for meeting these needs. She began working sporadically as a day laborer on local construction projects, cleaning newly installed windows and picking up debris. Her efforts earned her $7 per hour, a modest income that she did not report so as to avoid any hassle concerning her disability income. Indeed, many stable women devised clever strategies for meeting needs understood as only of "secondary" importance in the context of HIV services.

Charlotte, for example, was a savvy HIV/AIDS care consumer who devised a path to self-sufficiency, a destination she once knew well as a working-class home owner and career woman. Charlotte's career as a factory worker had been cut short by carpal tunnel syndrome and multiple injuries to various upper body muscles. When Charlotte was no longer able to work, she hit "rock bottom" due to her newly acquired addiction to cocaine. It wasn't until she lost her home in 1994 that Charlotte realized that she needed support. A friend explained to her that her injuries might make her eligible to receive disability benefits. In 1996 Charlotte's application for SSDI was approved. After living for a few years on "the bare minimum," Charlotte began "searching for a different future."

When I met Charlotte, she considered her daily life and health care needs in the context of her plans for future self-sufficiency. At the time of our first interview in 2008, she received approximately $950 per month. She also used multiple social programs such Housing Opportunities for People with AIDS (HOPWA), food stamps, and emergency assistance programs. She explained during an interview that the resources in Midway enabled her to make ends meet and "then some": "There are so many places that it will, like, overwhelm. It's so amazing. But that individual will have to go out and get it. It's not gonna just happen. . . . I have seen places where they'll bring your food. American Red Cross, they would come pick you up and take you to your doctor's appointment. So the resources are great in this area, the resources are great. Whether you dealing with medical bills or need some rent paid or a light bill paid, it is really here. If you go after it, you can have what you need."

Charlotte's awareness and use of area programs and resources for low-income individuals enabled her to live in relative comfort with few financial emergencies. However, she continued to identify and experience needs that stopped her from feeling as though she were self-sufficient. Updated clothing, salon visits, designer glasses, cosmetic dentistry, and gym memberships were just a few of the things she and other stable women identified as needs. They explained that their participation in consumer culture via shopping and social outings helped them to feel as though they were living life without HIV disease. Once women were freed from concentrating on how they would meet basic needs such as food and shelter, then they could begin addressing their social and emotional needs. Working toward living life as normally as possible was an important part of these women's emotional strategies for coping with the loss of income, the health crises, and the emotional burdens that often accompanied an HIV-positive diagnosis. Thus, for Charlotte, cosmetic dentistry was a pressing daily life need because her poor teeth affected her emotional balance and her prospects for long-term stability. As Charlotte described, "I can't be sitting here with a jacked-up mouth [crooked teeth]. My teeth are very important to me. People see your teeth, and when they look bad, they assume [you're] bad. When you look at your own teeth and they look bad, you feel bad about that first thing you present to the world—your face."

For Charlotte, dentistry was not just about oral health. It was a way to maintain a positive self-image and to project that image to others. Her image was important, given that her future plans included returning to school for professional certifications so that she could build a career as a substance abuse counselor. She hoped this career path would be personally fulfilling and conducive to reclaiming her place in "regular society." Charlotte thus slowly took on the financial burden of getting braces for her teeth. Straightening her teeth, though technically not considered a health need by Medicaid and Medicare programs, was important to her for emotional, social, and financial reasons. Had she enjoyed greater income or private insurance, her dentistry bills might not have been such a financial burden.

For stable women like Charlotte and Grace, income viability translated into housing stability. In short, they enjoyed better housing circumstances and prospects than their less stable counterparts. Charlotte, for example, lived in an apartment that was subsidized through the

HOPWA program. She described how she loved her apartment because it was in a beautiful neighborhood near a college campus. The yards were landscaped, the homes were historic, and her apartment blended in with the rest of the homes in the area. When asked if her rent was expensive, Charlotte responded, "No, my rent is based on my income. I pay about a hundred forty dollars a month. I live in one of the HOPWA housing [units]. Thank God for places that provide residences for people that are HIV-positive. It's just set up over there so that we can blend into the community. As far as people are concerned over there, it's another big, pretty house."

Charlotte appreciated that she had a subsidized apartment and lived in a "beautified neighborhood." She often said that the housing placement to which she was assigned was her "wildest dreams" come true. Charlotte also often spoke of wanting to own one of the homes in the neighborhood. She conceded that those particular homes were more than likely prohibitively expensive, but she still began to take the steps necessary for future home ownership. In 2006 Charlotte began saving for a home down payment. She worked with a local program for low- and medium-income individuals who want to be home owners that was designed to match the down payments of prospective buyers. She saved nearly $1,800 (the program's matching maximum for low-income families) over two years and was ready to explore the homes she would be able to afford with the matching payment. She found, however, that the homes for which she qualified were less than suitable. "I just refuse to live in a bad, drug-infested area. You know, if the house is there, I will still take it because I'm living in my house, I'm not living on the street. But if I have a choice in the matter, and I do have a choice, I'm not going to accept a house that it's in a bad, infested drug area. Because I have grandchildren. And their health and safety and well-being means everything to me as well as my own. So I have choices today."

By 2009 Charlotte had accessed vocational rehabilitation programs and had nearly completed the educational training and internship hours for her counseling certification. She felt confident that her prospective career, financial savings, and disability income would afford her a home and a future better than she had previously imagined for herself. All of her hard work also meant that she could qualify for a more expensive home because she could afford a greater mortgage. This prospective boost in her monthly income also meant that she would have to save more money to qualify for a medium-income matching grant. That summer she was enthusiastic about life. Unfortunately between 2009 and 2012, Charlotte experienced a few health-related financial setbacks. Her back injuries grew more painful, and as a result, she found it difficult to do the necessary studying for her certification exam. She also began experiencing short-term memory loss, a condition she attributed to stress and to the toxicity of HIV-related medications. Charlotte then turned to her plan B.

Being a programmatic services veteran of sorts, Charlotte searched for another program for permanent home ownership. She found Habitat for Humanity and quickly completed the application process. She decided to save the cash she had set aside for a down payment and, instead, built a line of "character credit" by volunteering her time and labor to building houses for other families in the program. Within fourteen months, Charlotte was granted a Habitat home of her own. She explained that

I started praying, and I said, "God, before long, I'm going to get a spot. Help me to be in a real good spot. A very quiet spot. I don't want to be in a spot where it's chaotic and drug trafficking." And I remember one lady, she told me, she said, "I have a community for you. You going to like it. You don't have any kids. It's a older community, and guess what, all of these homes are Habitat homes." So when I came, it was like I was right at home. And it's been a wonderful experience—they [social programs] allowed me to come in and just maneuver. I'm living out my dreams, man.

Stable women also experienced better housing prospects when relocating from one rental property to another. Joan and her husband, Michael, for example, enjoyed what they felt was desirable housing at the initiation of this study. They rented a small home in a middle-class subdivision on the outskirts of Midway. Joan and her husband together received $950 per month in ssdi and ssi payments. Joan was diagnosed as HIV-positive as a teenager, and early on, she experienced a serious bout of ill health and needed to access income-assistance programs.

Because of her abbreviated work history, she had not paid much into Social Security taxes, so Joan received only $327 per month. Although the combined $950 per month was well below the federal poverty line, their participation in the Section 8 housing program capped their monthly rental payments at $120. Joan's utility bills and lights were also subsidized through a Social Services energy assistance program available to low-income individuals. Joan and Michael paid only 30 percent of each month's total charges.

The $120 per month rent still afforded Joan a home that was welcoming and lush. Large trees, a green lawn, and small beds filled with flowers and vegetables greeted visitors. Joan was happy to report that although their home was small and old, it was pest free and in a safe neighborhood. All appliances worked, and Joan had even recently requested and received a new refrigerator from her landlord. As we sat in her living room well furnished with hand-me-downs, donated items, and "large ticket" items such as a big-screen television, Joan described why she enjoyed her house. "I lived in this house five years. I love this house. The rooms are nice and big. We have our own yard, a driveway—we don't have to fight for parking spaces. It's lovely. We have our own backyard. It's a old house, but it's a good house. It's in a good neighborhood, not a bad neighborhood. We don't really have to stress about anything there."

Joan discussed the house that she rented with Michael: It was well suited to their efforts to avoid stress. The house was large enough to accommodate their needs, including an outdoor patio that they dedicated to meditation and relaxation therapies. They lived in the house for five years and did not imagine that they would have any need to move, but then they felt the neighborhood began to decline.

Between 2009 and 2012 Joan and Michael operated a small, informal landscaping business for elderly and disabled residents in their neighborhood. They charged $20 to mow the lawn and weed any flower beds in need of care. For two summers they enjoyed a modest income boost that enabled them to have occasional "date nights" and make small upgrades to their home. The summer of 2011, however, ushered in residential change and, according to Joan, "the wrong kind of neighbors." The death of two elderly residents on the block left two homes on the rental market. When Joan and Michael introduced themselves to the new tenants, they at first felt they had found friends. Not long after Joan offered the new tenants their lawn care services. Soon, however, someone broke into her toolshed and stole the lawnmower. Throughout that summer, Joan dealt with various types of vandalism to her property: uprooted plants, a broken mailbox, and, once, a broken window. She blamed the new tenants because they had proven themselves "loud and just the jealous type. They didn't like us making money and doing okay." That fall Joan began searching for a new home.

By the time we met again in 2012, Joan and Michael had moved into a new apartment. Joan loved her new apartment because it was clean, spacious, and quiet. The couple enjoyed amenities such as big windows, a swimming pool, exercise facilities, and nearby bus lines and bike trails leading to two different shopping plazas. To put it simply, Joan felt the move "was a blessing because they actually [got us] more [amenities] for basically the same money."

Joan's relative material comfort was supported by her social networking strategy. In contrast to vulnerable women who tried (sometimes to the detriment of their physical safety) to maintain as many operative network members as possible, stable women honed their personal support networks to include service professionals and financially and emotionally stable friends. Their abilities to maintain these friendships with service professionals and similarly positioned individuals were possible because stable women could participate in activities such as occasionally dining out and going to the movies.

Stable women also honed their personal networks by disconnecting from members who used drugs or who were insensitive about HIV disease. Women such as Joan who had never dealt with chemical dependency issues did not necessarily go through the process of "shrinking" their networks. However, those women who had traveled the roads of recovery did go through the process of letting go of old social patterns and networks. They could afford to do so because they had a kind of financial and social security that vulnerable women did not. Any associates, friends, and acquaintances who might have been part of women's past lives as drug users, drinkers, or dangers to themselves could be and, for all practical purposes, were left behind. DeeDee explained, "I don't have a lot of friends. Friends get you in trouble. You know what my grandmama always told me? 'If you buy a person a plant, if that plant lives, that's a true friend. If it dies,' she said, 'run like hell. They mean you no good.' And a lot of friends is like that when you out there using drugs."

DeeDee's remark that "friends get you in trouble" comes from hard-learned experience during the times when she was in active drug addiction. Her lack of friends in the present context was a strategy for avoiding the trouble that can accompany drug use and addiction. Charlotte similarly explained her lack of close friends during the time of this research: "It depend on the person; if you're not on real good solid ground, it is in your best interest to leave the idea of any friends behind. Because drug addiction is very powerful, and people will get you back to using and involved in a cycle quicker than you can clean. So, like, I don't try to go out there and convert nobody or try to persuade them to stop using. You don't even hang with them anymore."

Like other women who had achieved long-term recovery, Charlotte and DeeDee chose to leave old friends behind to prevent the possibility of a future drug use relapse. Other women also disconnected from friends when they felt they couldn't trust them to keep their HIV status a secret. This situation meant that stable women, compared to other women in this study, relied most heavily upon programmatic services to meet their needs, a strategy that, as I explore in the following chapter, their relative economic and social stability enabled.

As the women's circumstances attest, all of the women in this study struggled to make ends meet each month. The types of material needs study participants struggled with, however, varied according to the daily life conditions under which they strove for stability and financial security. In this chapter I've detailed the variability of living conditions among the study participants, and it provides a means of more finely considering their support service needs. The disaggregation of this public health population makes clear that some women struggled to afford food, find basic shelter, and keep themselves safe from assault while others struggled to find suitable long-term housing, pay monthly utility bills, and abstain from illicit drug use. Still other women struggled to afford material wants, or needs made ponderable by relative economic security. In all instances, however, it was the confluence of economic factors that shaped the varied realities of women's lives. A generic one-size-fits-all explanation of client needs and circumstances hardly expresses the multiple and context-specific needs the HIV-positive women encountered in relation to maintaining their health. Indeed, unpacking the label "client" as it related to low-income Black women highlights the importance of the subtle details of these women's lives that social service guidelines and service protocols often left unaddressed.

Ultimately these patterns of social difference provide the micro-contextual lens through which I magnify and render visible the women's varied journeys along the pathways of inequality blighting the terrains of the Ryan White CARE Act. In the following chapters, I elaborate how conditions of socioeconomic difference mattered for women living with HIV/AIDS in terms of their service use strategies and their access to support. Structuring this analysis in light of intra-population difference highlights an enduring need to critically interrogate public health parlance and practice, which have historically viewed HIV-positive Black women as a more or less homogenous group characterized by a shared experience of poverty, race, and gender.

4 The Pedagogy of Policy Reform

> Education either functions as an instrument which is used to
> facilitate integration of the younger generation into the logic of
> the present system and bring about conformity or it becomes the
> practice of freedom, the means by which men and women deal
> critically and creatively with reality and discover how to participate
> in the transformation of their world.
>
> PAULO FREIRE, *Pedagogy of the Oppressed*

The complicated details of women's lives shaped their abilities to adapt to changes in Midway's system of care. New programs, changes in eligibility rules to federal and state programs, and revised agency-specific guidelines for using services threatened to revoke the eligibility of even the most seasoned HIV/AIDS care veterans. Community leaders, however, seemed to interpret "client grumbling," as some called it, as issues of distrust for new employees and frustration with "having to do more for their benefits." This ultimately framed the clients' experiences in terms of their individual emotional states rather than in terms related to their varied structural positions within the system. To help ease what were perceived as the "growing pains" of changes in services, clients and care providers were presented a variety of mostly optional, if strongly recommended, programs and workshops. Perhaps largely for practical purposes, a series of HIV/AIDS-related educational forums was implemented alongside the newly elaborated suite of services. I refer to these forums as the "pedagogy of HIV/AIDS care" because they represent a series of formal educational venues through which care recipients and service providers were taught how to think about HIV/AIDS and their roles, rights, and responsibilities as participants in the system of care.

In *Pedagogy of the Oppressed*, Paolo Freire (2000) asserts that education is a dichotomous enterprise: it can facilitate domination or it can be used to liberate the oppressed. While I partially frame my interpretation of Midway's system of care through the critical lens of Freire's theory of pedagogy, I also struggle with his notion that educational systems are "either/or" operations. For example, I can see how public health interventions constitute a particular manner of teaching that often acculturates target populations to rules and values of the predominant social and moral order. Horton and Barker (2009), in this way, highlight public health discourses and intervention practices as central to contemporary practices of race making, subjectivity, and social exclusion. They argue that oral public health campaigns in California enlist migrant farmworkers in an instrument of governance, providing a rich site for constructions of deservingness and social belonging. Deservingness in this setting, they maintain, is based on an individual's conformity with commonly held hygienic practices and biomedical values related to self-governance. Certainly, as I demonstrate in coming chapters, the Ryan White CARE Act's suite of programs is no exception to the use of public health programs as a tool for enculturation; it is, after all, an arm of the American body of governance. Yet when seen from women's diverse vantage points in Midway's public system of HIV/AIDS care, the lessons taught under the rubric of Ryan White legislation defy easy characterization as either "liberating" or "oppressive." As Ong (1995) reminds us in the public health care context of refugee medicine, power is dispersed between individuals and social groups. The HIV/AIDS care recipients and providers engaged with the public health care structures in strategic ways and to various ends. It turned out that sometimes lessons taught in this HIV/AIDS care context worked to the women's advantage; however, at other times, they placed the women at great disadvantage. The key to discerning power in this setting as "dispersed" was to understand how educational goals achieved objectives of governance while, at the same time, the women drew from, resisted, and/or transformed those goals to meet their specific needs. To put it simply, women were not powerless in this system.

This chapter explains key lessons of the Ryan White reauthorization legislation as it was implemented in Midway through a series of educational programs designed to increase the women's fluency with the values of personal responsibility. In reaction to fiscal oversight measures and the medicalization of the Ryan White CARE Act, the general service provider community sought to safeguard local Ryan White CARE Act programs from a perceived threat of future disinvestment by redoubling efforts to create model care consumers. In 2008 as Emily, a former executive director of Health Partnership put it, "The Ryan White Modernization Act actually sunsets next year, but they're probably going to do continuation funding on it for three more years. Now within that, and after that, there's the real potential for them to cap how much we can spend on any one service or any one client. That's just a reality, assuming that they will not add enough new money at the legislative level."

In a context of future uncertainty, Health Partnership staff sought to ensure compliance with federal directives "by weeding out the riffraff," as one care provider explained, and excluding from services those individuals who did not conform to expectations of behavior change and self-management. Because federal legislation prioritized medical care and behavioral change programs conducive to medical compliance, care recipients were counseled as conditions of service eligibility to try abstention from illicit drug use, to attain regular medical care, to adhere to medication regimens as prescribed, and to strive for financial stability. Self-management was indeed a key feature of Health Partnership's specific service provision strategy and of the broader HIV-related service provider community more generally.

Increased policy emphasis on oversight and medical programs paradoxically enlisted Health Partnership employees in this medium of governance as both subjects and instruments of power. In other words, policy changes in the Ryan White program had the effect of shaping Health Partnership employees into agents of the state who imposed a rigid set of ideas on those who came for help. In some cases employees felt powerless to do much of anything else. Policy reform thus created both model consumers *and* providers of HIV/AIDS care. The implication was that Ryan White programs could create care providers and consumers who would "move forward" to realize the future promise, respectfully, of managing the epidemic well and of living their lives healthfully. The study participants' involvement in the CARE Act continuum thus included expectations of behavior change in ways that were protective of institutional viability while under broader conditions of social services decline (Carr 2011; Nguyen 2010).

Discipline and Care Provision

Care providers were obliged to attend state-sponsored workshops and training sessions as conditions of their employment. One of the most notable workshops I attended involved training to use CAREWare, a free software program designed to manage data derived from clinical care and support services for people living with HIV/AIDS. CAREWare was distributed by HRSA, and the state of North Carolina mandated its use. Care providers at different organizations especially valued the software because they could network their case files, theoretically enabling physicians and support service providers to see a "fuller" picture of an individual's health-related needs and challenges. It would also reduce referral duplication and increase the services' efficiency by making it possible for care providers to share and request information instantaneously. Every client entered into the CAREWare database would be automatically tracked by any participating organization that served that client.

Service providers could also easily produce service reports that would allow the state consortium and the federal government to quickly assess statistics of programmatic services use. CAREWare tracked how many clients particular organizations served and the particular types of services they used. It also tracked the money disbursed and from which particular contract the money came. When the entirety of funds from a particular contract had been spent, service providers were unable to enter the service. This prevented organizations and the state from overspending relative to federal grant award amounts.

Perhaps the most important feature of CAREWare, however, was the volume of information it required and housed about individual clients. Gone were the days when care providers could quickly assess needs and complete paperwork for funds disbursement. Gone too were the days of filing incomplete paperwork or of strategically not documenting certain details about clients' lives. Each client file required several fields of information before any application for assistance could be viewed as complete. CAREWare not only collected data such as case management notes, services provided, and the amount of funds disbursed, but it also provided a virtual forum for disseminating clinical information such as prescribed medication regimens, clinical diagnoses, mental health and substance abuse assessments, and laboratory diagnostics. CAREWare supplied a venue for tracking triglyceride and glucose levels and screenings for hepatitis B, tuberculosis, syphilis, chlamydia, human papillomavirus, and gonorrhea. Most important it verified regular participation in medical care by storing results obtained from the CD4 cell counts and viral load testing that were required as a condition of using services. For care providers the CAREWare workshop made material and explicit the policy concern with fiscal oversight and, by extension, the methods by which care providers determined service eligibility. Care providers, in turn, learned to manage their daily activities and service encounters in the regimented ways that the software required. They were in effect disciplined in the Foucaultian (1978) sense of having their behaviors, activities, and timetables regimented by Ryan White policy. For example, Emily explained,

> [the government] want[s] to be able to track who's getting the money, how it's getting used, and how it affects health outcomes. It's that health outcome link, you know. Prove what your t-cell count is now and what it was a year ago and what we did for you in between. . . . The paperwork, as you know, there's more and more of it every single year. We started off with one little page that we created internally, and it turned into three pages, and then it was ten. And now it just goes on and on, that whole government requirement. I guess that's because we're all just terrified that our taxpayers' dollars are going to be stolen.

As Emily said, oversight measures encompassed by the state adoption of CAREWare potentially demonstrated services efficacy as well as honesty in client and care provider dealings with federal money. The implicit concern was that in the absence of clearly articulated and closely monitored service provision protocol, clients and/or care providers would have spent funds inappropriately. This implicit presumption of inappropriate behavior was also reinforced during community-wide educational forums.

Community Events as Pedagogical Exercise

Educational forums and annual treatment update conferences organized by local care providers and HIV-related institutions provided two formal venues where clients and support service providers were taught to reinforce values of self-management and personal responsibility. For example, Midway's annual treatment update conference focused on facilitating dialogue between medical practitioners and their HIV-positive patients. The forum was specifically designed as a means through which doctors and representatives from clinical trials could communicate advances in treatment and care. The local Community Advisory Board organized and facilitated the meeting.[1] When I attended the meeting in 2008, representatives of clinical trials emphasized the relatively quick and impressive advances that had been made in HIV/AIDS treatment. Since the days of AZT therapy, twenty-eight new drugs had been developed for managing HIV disease and preventing the onset of AIDS. Viral load, medication resistance testing, and CD4 cell counts—all also tracked patient responses to HIV infection and progress with therapy. The clinical trials community was happy to announce that over the past year, three new drugs had been approved for the treatment of HIV infection.[2] New drugs offered hope for individuals with resistant strains of the virus as well as for individuals with complicated or physically cumbersome medication regimens. The keynote speaker explained, "The drug research continues to come down the pike. We will likely see more of these advances as time goes on. Be sure to talk to your doctors and explore what options might be right for you." Although the explicit goal of the update was to inform consumers about recent developments in HIV/AIDS treatment protocol, it also invited program participants to entertain the notion of future treatment protocol changes and to identify and act on their own health care needs. Thus in addition to the official treatment update, this particular forum also served as a platform for advocating particular aspects of self-managed care. The notion of self-management, or taking personal responsibility for one's health, was further developed by the topical themes of guest speakers who were brought in to complement the clinical trials reporting.

For example, a lay guest speaker focused on communicating what he described as "his message of adherence." He explained that statistically, as a gay White man who was diagnosed in 1984, he should not have been alive. He owed his success as a twenty-four-year survivor, he said, to his diligent efforts to build a life around the notion of adherence. After more than a decade of "living one day at a time," he continued, "it's possible to have long-term goals now." The speaker related his experience of survival to certain subjects such as his returning to work, his volunteerism in the HIV-positive community, and his responsibility to build a support team. Physicians, case managers, pharmacists, peers, family, and friends, he explained, should all be rallied in support of one's health care and maintenance. It meant building positive, working relationships "based on the needs and accomplishments of the patient." The speaker further urged HIV-positive individuals to keep track of their own viral loads, CD4 cell counts, and medication side effects. These efforts, he argued, were the keys to thriving in what he had come to think of as "an adventure in possibilities."

A physician continued the focus on medication adherence and personal responsibility for health and spoke about the importance of behavioral intervention for maximizing the benefits of HIV health care. She asked program participants to assess their own risk for "ineffectively using" health care resources: "Do you follow medications as prescribed? Do you inform all of your doctors about changes in medication? Do you use condoms, share needles, or donate blood or breast milk?" The presumption was that if an individual answered any of her questions incorrectly, she or he had stopped short of realizing the benefits of public health care eligibility by possibly failing to stop disease progression and/or viral transmission. In all three talks given that day, speakers prompted audience members to conceive of HIV health as an individual achievement or failure to manage one's health-related responsibilities.

Another conference designed for the local HIV-positive community reinforced ideals of self-management in relation to a perceived eminent decline in Ryan White funding for support services. The conference was organized and hosted by several local agencies, including Health Partnership, the North Carolina of Department of Health, and the state's Ryan White consortium. The keynote speaker, a noted HIV/AIDS activist and public health scholar, introduced ideals of individualism and personal responsibility, imploring HIV-positive individuals to "take control" of their lives, their health care, and their role in changing public perceptions concerning HIV disease. "You have to be responsible for yourself before you can be responsible for anyone else," he reasoned. The speaker defined "being responsible for oneself" through vignettes concerning adherence to medical treatment directives and abstention from illicit drug use. He highlighted the usefulness of compliance with behavioral norms in service settings. And he urged conference attendees to disprove negative public perceptions of HIV-positive individuals by exhibiting a "public self" who defies negative stereotypes. "Be a little better than you were yesterday," he said. "Reduce the number and impact of negative influences in your life." He closed his address by lamenting the "planned shrinkage" of housing and financial support programs for HIV-positive populations. He asserted that the loss of state funding for support programs would be seen as inappropriate only when HIV-positive individuals were seen as "worthy" of support.

After the address, conference attendees attended workshops on self-care, spiritual support, sexual health, and/or treatment adherence. I attended a women's-only workshop along with several HIV-positive research participants I had come to know through my fieldwork. This particular workshop was an offshoot of Health Partnership's support group for women, "Living Life Golden," a weekly discussion group designed to teach effective strategies for living well with HIV disease. The facilitator began the workshop by explaining the need for "self-acceptance and love as we live our lives": "The self is a vehicle, and we need to begin the process of moving forward." She urged women to move forward in their lives by adopting "healthy strategies for resisting control by others who don't want what's best for you." Throughout the workshop, the facilitator introduced "barriers to well-being" such as a fixation on things beyond one's control, poor communication skills, low self-esteem, and self-destructive coping mechanisms such as drug use. She implored workshop participants to engage in service use strategies that would create positive working relationships and facilitate well-being:

speaking quietly, attending appointments as scheduled, asking for (rather than demanding) help, and accepting responsibility for "those things we can control" while letting go of "what we cannot." The workshop organizer emphasized the women's personal capacities to modify their behavior, reminding everyone that "if we come to an appointment with attitude, we will be met with attitude."

At the end of the meeting, the facilitator distributed aluminum "wedding bands" and asked us each to "commit" to ourselves by taking a pledge of empowerment. Prompting us to place the rings on our fingers, she asked us to repeat, "I promise to know myself and to communicate respect for myself and for others. I love me enough. I'm going to do everything I need to take care of my body." At the end of the pledge, she pronounced us all "officially empowered and wed to [ourselves]."

These community events and workshops provided important vehicles for disseminating techniques of self-management such as social deference and self-initiated treatment change. Although public workshops and speeches conveyed useful skills for navigating interpersonal dimensions of client-provider relationships, the focus on the particular highlighted themes suggested that some individuals deserved the poor health care outcomes they experienced; moreover, the tenor of the events also encouraged the clients' docility. Suggested survival strategies embodied neoliberal values of deservedness, self-regulation, and individualism in the sense that they shifted the onus for access to health care and basic needs from the state to the individual. In the process the women were conditioned to use their bodies and speech as instruments for conveying consonance with personal responsibility. The pedagogical implication was that those women who did not "perform" in ways that reflected these values would encounter obstacles to care. In later chapters I call such performances of these emotional styles "using 'survival' to survive" because they represent ideologically driven but pragmatic means by which the women could maximize their access to resources (see also Carr 2011). By communicating their consonance with the values of survival in the post-TMA era, the women secured daily life resources and, in some cases, the means for their upward mobility. This particular "emotional style" of requesting and receiving services became an important, if informal, criterion for service eligibility among service providers struggling with policy-given oversight measures (Hochschild 2003, 5).

Agency-Level Pedagogical Exercises

Given a macro-level and community-wide emphasis on behavior change as a prerequisite for medical compliance, Health Partnership employees had a common understanding of the pedagogical requirements of their jobs. Health Partnership staff transformed policy-driven, community-wide lessons of survival into agency-administered rules and service provision goals. Like welfare workers more generally, public HIV/AIDS health care providers in Midway were charged with the vague task of transforming policy mandates for efficiency and fiscal restraint into self-management strategies that the poor could put into practice (Morgen, Acker, and Weigt 2010). Indeed, Health Partnership's unofficial view of the TMA was that its primary objective was fiscal reform rather than health. As one care provider explained, the TMA "is not patient-centered. And they don't do anything in terms of the public focus on health. They're just ridiculous oversights that say, 'We control the money, and we don't want to pay your rent anymore.' Never mind that without rent you will be homeless and probably get very sick." This interpretation of the TMA reflected a general, if not critical, appreciation for the systematic dismantling of the HIV/AIDS safety net. When prompted to further explain the agency's perspective on the policy, Greg explained that the TMA was aimed at "teaching responsibility to people who are used to getting something for nothing." In other words, care providers at Health Partnership understood HIV/AIDS care policy changes in relation to the discourse of deservingness, even if they personally disagreed with it.

Health Partnership employees additionally operated under a related concern for the financial survival of Health Partnership, a concern directly related to the existence of their jobs as well as resources for the poor and HIV-positive. Given the importance of these issues, employees were well versed in a logic positing how agency funding was correlated with the appropriate provision and use of services. In other words, the pedagogy of personal responsibility was a key service provision goal because it ensured the continuation of Health Partnership programs. Case manager Natasha explained that "the money that comes to us has

[to] be used appropriately, or we won't be fed. I'm listening to the person that holds the food. I'm new to this town, but I'm not new to Ryan White. . . . If you want these doors to stay open, you have to show you are making the changes so eventually you don't need us."

"Appropriate" services provision and use were related to goals of self-management and behavior change. In turn, appropriate services use could theoretically enable clients to create for themselves conditions of "a life well lived," or survival beyond the bare fact of living. Bert further described the pedagogical requirements of his job:

> It [appropriate services provision] has to do with teaching a client to do things for themselves like filling out an application for a job. . . . You may have a hard time not doing it for them, but you can't. Sometimes little things like that make them so dependent on us. . . . We have to go through our cases to see who is in need of [financial support], who is showing that they can handle it. Who's struggling to make it, enduring, sustaining compliance? Are they doing the right thing? Are they staying in compliance with medical treatment, following up with appointments here, and are they maybe looking for a job or maybe in school?

And Natasha outlined hers:

> My goal as a case manager is to make clients self-sufficient. Making them accountable for their actions—"Yes, I may have been practicing unsafe sex, but after I found that I was positive, I had to change that action. I love having sex, but now I'm having a condom each time I'm loving having sex." I'm not telling them to stop the lifestyle; it's just trying to teach them how to alter the lifestyle that will allow them to continue having a lifetime. And, with that, I tell the client, "Once you get to the point where you don't need me, it's okay. You don't need me for the rest of your life." It's there for a cushion but not a crutch.

As providers such as Natasha and Bert well understood, teaching clients skills of self-management was inherent to federal and state expectations of oversight and therapeutic change. Teaching clients to be personally responsible, in other words, ensured the integrity of this branch of a social safety net, a human services arm that was increasingly scrutinized as morally suspect and economically costly. "If [they] are not helping their self and [we] continue paying for them, we are helping them use or abuse the system," Bert explained. In turn, clients would potentially become used to receiving "something for nothing" and would feel "entitled" to services that were otherwise discretionary. Providers such as Natasha explained that "entitlement" referred to the attitude that "'because I am [HIV]-positive, I'm entitled to everything.' This feeling of entitlement is crazy. You know? I'm sorry historically you've been able to walk through this door and get services upon your beck and call, but this is not Burger King and you don't get it your way. . . . You have responsibilities that I have to enforce."

As Natasha explained, Health Partnership employees understood entitlement as an attitude antithetical to personal responsibility. Entitled clients expected support based on their HIV-positive status rather than on their conformity with the value of personal responsibility and the practice of self-management. Yet as representatives of the state and the HIV-positive community more generally, Health Partnership employees were obligated to use public funds in the most effective and fair way possible. In light of their responsibilities to counsel individual clients on behavior management, to protect the fiscal health of the organization, and to further public health goals, employees saw entitled attitudes in a negative light. Consider what Keith further said about entitlement: "A lot of clients think—most clients think they're entitled to things. I don't think they know about eligibility. . . . You know, 'we may be able to help you if you meet the certain criteria' as opposed to 'all right, since you're HIV-positive, you're guaranteed to get everything we have to offer.' I think a lot of clients feel entitled and don't even try to show the right attitude."

Keith described a common understanding among Health Partnership service providers: the majority of clients assumed that support resources were theirs for the taking without stipulations. However, increased oversight in the TMA circumscribed staff attempts to regulate how and why clients accessed financial support services.[3] Put bluntly, care providers were indeed aware that the TMA policy was aimed at disciplining them. The behaviors and actions of agency employees were regulated by policy pronouncements requiring fiscal oversight and restricted redistribution of state-sponsored resources. Care providers thus strove to meet their clients' needs in ways that were respectful of federal rules and guidelines. Providers focused much of their attention on counseling about behavior change, documenting progress in behaviors, and providing referrals to educational workshops. Throughout this research, care providers advised the women to attend a broad range of workshops, including the previously described forums, financial counseling classes sponsored by vocational rehabilitation services, nutritional education workshops sponsored by Health Partnership, and an informational session designed and facilitated by a college intern about how to use coupons.

Over the course of five years, the women were offered, prompted, and sometimes outright cajoled into participating in an educational system designed to facilitate their effective use of public health care resources. As study participants learned the rules and expectations of services provision and use in the post-TMA era, they joined a moral economy based on a notion of survival infused with American values of personal responsibility. The pedagogical exercises of Midway's system of care helped the women to understand how to help themselves in a changing material and ideological landscape.

However, the HIV-positive women highlighted in this study were not simply subjected to the logic of HIV-related education in the Foucaultian (1978) sense of training their actions. The HIV-related educational system was not monolithically oppressive. Some women strategized for access to resources using their capacity for subjection and, by drawing on that capacity, asserted their belonging in a moral economy of HIV/AIDS care organized around the notion of personally responsible survivorship.

In chapters 5 and 6, I examine this particular notion of survival as a cultural resource consisting of two interlocking components—personal responsibility and biomedical consonance. As a concept defined and used by public health care providers in relation to programmatic services efficiency and laboratory diagnostics, survival offered women a blueprint for navigating the socially exclusive terrains of the HIV/AIDS-related social safety net. In this sense, the women's HIV-positive status, when combined with appropriate performances of survival, potentially offered them a means of claiming access to state resources that otherwise were in decline. This kind of biologically mediated social inclusion was, however, contingent on local conditions and processes.

As Guell (2011), Marsland (2012), and Marsland and Prince (2012) remind us, social belonging organized around disease diagnosis is complex and fragmented. In other words, a shared diagnosis of HIV disease does not necessarily mean that the women in this study also shared identities, experiences, or practices. Other aspects of social life and the women's specific life circumstances stifled some of their claims to citizenship and support while privileging those of others. The following chapters thus examine differences in the women's abilities to convey their conformity with the pedagogical exercises associated with survival to more broadly consider contingencies of biosocial inclusion in U.S. federally funded HIV/AIDS care.

5. Using "Survival" to Survive, Part I

> Why would I want to focus on challenges or disappointment? What
> good does that do me? It's about being thankful for what you got.
>
> LADY E., an HIV-positive woman

During my first formal interview with Lady E., she emphasized how
"blessed" she was in life. I was confused because she had already shared
with me some of the obstacles she faced for well-being. In the less formal spaces of the Health Partnership waiting room and the bus stop,
she had discussed conditions of poverty and drug addiction recovery as
topping the list of her daily concerns. Throughout our first interview,
however, she skillfully avoided my prompts to discuss details of her life's
challenges in depth. "Why now," I wondered, "would she refuse to speak
of the challenges she faces?" I initially assumed her refusal to speak in
what I defined as candid terms was the result of a lack of trust and, possibly, discomfort with the formal interview process; certainly, those
conditions mattered here. However, I had also yet to realize at this early
stage of my research that Lady E.'s initial refusal to speak of hardship
was part of a service use strategy that the changing material and ideological landscape of federally funded HIV/AIDS care made necessary.

My field notes frequently describe how she sat in the lobby of Health
Partnership, crocheting baby booties and hats out of pastel yarn that a
neonatal unit in a nearby hospital supplied to her. Most of the time she
waited upward of an hour before the agency counselors with whom she
had regularly scheduled appointments could see her. Many clients complained long before they had waited an hour. Others simply left. Yet
Lady E. waited patiently, typically remaining silent and steadfast in her
work. With her legs crossed at her ankles and her shoulders and face

lowered to her hands, she passed the time seemingly unaffected by the chaotic bustle of agency staff and the clients they served. I often wondered how she remained focused and calm amid the clamor of nearby client–service provider disagreements, the constantly ringing telephone, and the jarring buzz of the front door's electronic lock system. I initially assumed she had been desensitized to the sounds of the building and the squabbles between clients in need of support and care providers in need of documentation for those support requests. Over time I realized, however, Lady E. was none of those things.

I eventually learned to see Lady E.'s calm demeanor in a new light. She was not quiet but selective about with whom she "shared her business." She was also not impervious to her surroundings. To the contrary, she was sensitive to her surroundings to the extent that she took to managing her anxiety by focusing her attention on crochet work and, later, on beading. Neither was it true that she was desensitized to the charged atmosphere of an underfunded HIV/AIDS service organization in a city hit hard by the epidemic. What I much later figured out was that Lady E., in her words, had learned the strategic "importance of being thankful" for what she had.

Throughout my work in Midway, women such as Lady E. faced life challenges and hardships I have been privileged enough to avoid. Stories of homelessness, violence, addiction, ill health, neglect, and social isolation are interwoven throughout my field notes and interview transcripts. Yet also present are statements of gratitude, accounts of life-affirming experiences, and stories that show an appreciation of the value of small gestures, good intentions, and the ability to draw on inner strength. "These," I wrote in my field notes, "are stories of survival—stories of vulnerability, adaptation, and perseverance." I admired, and still do, the women's courageous efforts to live well and claim happiness amid formidable barriers to health and well-being. I was right, I think, to feel as though these women were teaching me something of survivorship in the particular sense of acting in a social world that denied the realities of their struggle. Undoubtedly these stories were of that kind of coping. Yet as I illuminate in the following pages, these stories were also about how women demonstrated behavior change goals embedded in the TMA by using survival as a cultural resource. Sometimes the women skillfully used gratitude and appreciation, locally valued sentiments associated with survival discourse in the post-TMA era. In this sense the women's stories of survival told the tale of how they endeavored to act *on* a social world whose gatekeepers were trained to question their right to be in it.

In this chapter I focus specifically on the women's efforts to prove their consonance with fiscally driven values of personal responsibility. I draw on Bourdieu's (1986) notion of "social capital," a concept referring to collective resources and/or benefits produced and obtained through institutionalized networks of reciprocity. The term "social capital" allows me to emphasize how social relationships with care providers and tools of neoliberalism structured the women's abilities to advance their own social and economic interests. Chase (2011) explores a similar dynamic among Latinas navigating public HIV/AIDS care in New Jersey. She explains that familiarity with middle-class knowledge of bureaucracy and norms of comportment operate as social leverage for women trying to build diversely populated networks of HIV-related support. "The more diverse the network," Chase points out, "the more different kinds of resources can be derived from it" (2011, 18). In this sense I use social capital as a way to understand the women's agency in an institutional context thick with behavioral prescriptions, unequal social relationships, and disempowering narratives of dependency and individualism. I argue that through discourses and behaviors commensurate with personal responsibility, the women sought and sometimes obtained advantages in the public HIV/AIDS care system. Thus I use social capital as a means to focus on the reality that study participants made deliberate choices in their social relationships and programmatic service journeys. Women were not merely passive recipients of aid and health care services (Maternowska 2006); to the contrary, they were tactical and sometimes savvy participants in the institutional settings mediating their lives and health.

Important to note, however, is that Bourdieu's social capital concept does not focus on how uneven terrains of material life may engender novel forms of social advantage and exclusion in a given social milieu. His conception suggests that social capital is a "durable resource" because it is more or less entrenched in the social structures circumscribing group membership (Bourdieu 1986, 248). In other words, for Bourdieu, social capital represents a benefit to be acquired and possessed through never-ending efforts to secure institutionalized advantages. Understood in this way, the social capital concept fails to fully account for transformation in conditions and advantages of group membership. It is an end-point rather than a process actively negotiated and defined by actors who may be vying for acknowledgement and recognition from diverse material positions. In this sense social capital cannot fully encompass the women's experiences with health policy and programmatic service changes because it cannot account for what circumscribes material and social advantages of moral membership in the American social safety net. It also cannot fully account for the novelty of the women's strategies for transforming otherwise contingent social relations into more durable networks of advantage.

For this reason I suggest the women's transformations and their use of social capital in this context to be understood in relation to the notion of "social network surrogacy," or the processes through which the women associated with service professionals and organizations in order to generate beneficial social and economic ties. In a context wherein kinship and neighborhood ties were weak and/or overburdened, the women found new ways of asserting solidarity with their care providers and, in turn, of compelling them to provide various forms of financial and psychosocial support. These relationships, however, were typically provisional and temporary as the policies and protocol of Health Partnership always circumscribed and at least partially delimited them. While individual service professionals wielded discretionary power to disburse or withhold benefits, the institution ultimately allocated the aid that the women sought. The benefits of social capital within the milieu of federally funded HIV/AIDS care thus remained situational, substitutive, and thus surrogate in nature.

Stable Women and Social Network Surrogacy

In general the system of care operated beneficially for women who created and maintained ties of obligation and/or trust with programmatic service employees. This difficult undertaking required time, resources, and the understanding and use, if not internalization, of various facets of personal responsibility. Stable women excelled at network building, and, in a practical sense, Health Partnership employees described them as embodying the best of what HIV/AIDS care offered. They were at various times referred to as "agency success stories" and/ or "easy to help." That they were easy to help was evident by the social standards to which they adhered and by which they were partly defined. They set the bar, so to speak, and modeled for care providers how personal responsibility for one's health could be proven by performances of gratitude and moral uprightness, "appropriate" service use patterns, and volunteerism. Each of these strategies had the effect of communicating the stable women's social distance from the general population of clients, a group that service professionals sometimes openly maligned.

It is perhaps no surprise that of the nine women considered here as stable, seven were "regulars" at the community events described in chapter 4. Indeed, community events were an important part of stable women's social network strategies as attendance provided them with a means for talking with support service professionals apart from their assistance requests and services protocol. Community events were generally happy occasions that care providers and the women usually enjoyed as a day away from predictable routines of daily life. In addition to educational lectures and activities facilitating behavior change, community events typically included catered food; a steady supply of coffee, sodas, and juice; music from a deejay; and a raffle that included coveted prizes such as iPods and gift cards to Wal-Mart.

While client-provider relations were not totally redefined in these settings, they were less formal and more playful than what I had observed at Health Partnership. Providers and clients went outside to smoke together at breaks, oftentimes sharing personal and humorous stories about their families or opinions about popular news or television programming. Sharing lunch and recreational time also created a heightened sense of familiarity among community members. After all only in this type of setting did care providers have the opportunity to witness and admire, for example, how much sixty-eight-year-old Danielle loved to dance. And only in this type of setting could Danielle have experienced firsthand Greg's "mad skills" as a DJ. Under these circumstances, stable women and care providers perhaps learned to appreciate one another anew as individuals with endearing social qualities.

Even still the core of the women's advantages in the HIV/AIDS health care system was their ability to put pedagogical lessons of behavior change into practice. Their performance of gratitude provided one means by which women could convey their personal responsibility for their lives and health. Personal responsibility in part referred to the women's individual recognition that they should look only to themselves for economic stability and advancement. Gratitude, in this context, provided a means for the women to distance themselves from negative stereotypes concerning the poor attitudes of ungrateful "others." Stable women dissociated themselves from less favored clients by vocalizing their gratitude and mindfulness concerning how "lucky" they were to receive assistance. Stacey, for example, was a stable woman who had maintained long-term sobriety. When I met her, she was three years sober, but she chose to continue living in a substance abuse recovery facility designed for women recently released from voluntary and court-mandated state-supported detoxification programs. Essentially Stacey lived in a rooming house with several other women who were variably motivated to work with their recovery programs. Despite enjoying amenities of life in a suburban neighborhood, Stacey described living in the rooming house as "sometimes hard" because she had little privacy. Her fellow residents often listened as she talked on the phone. It made Stacey especially nervous because she feared an accidental disclosure of her HIV status would lead to ridicule and isolation. She made a habit of talking on the phone outside, even during cold winter months, and kept her prescription medications hidden in the top of her bedroom closet. Even so, one woman learned Stacey's secret and began to tease her in front of the other residents. Stacey lamented on two separate occasions how one of her housemates tactlessly asked her, "How freaky was you that you got that shit?"

Stacey also acknowledged the stress she felt as a woman determined to stay clean while living among women in various stages of sobriety. According to Stacey, the mood of the house was "intense" because some occupants didn't really want to be there while other occupants were absorbed in the emotionally difficult work of "owning their past mistakes."[1] Persistent conflict between individual women was made worse by the reality that drug use frequently occurred in the recovery house, despite its therapeutic purpose. Some women snuck drugs inside and, more commonly, returned from off-site group meetings apparently high. Yet even in these undesirable conditions, Stacey reported that she was "lucky." Asked what she meant by being lucky, she explained: "I have no expectations because I feel like—because the life that I led—all that stuff to me is, like, it's good. I really don't be expecting nothing. . . . I'm just glad [Health Partnership is] there to help at all."

Stacey did not expect assistance because she was a former drug user. Presumably her former drug use meant that she was undeserving of help in the present. Her stigmatized identity as an addict spoiled her right to expect support for basic human needs such as food and shelter. Any support she did receive, however modest, was good because she had no social rights to any of it.

Now that she was in recovery, however, Stacey turned her "undeserving" status into an advantage by which she could solicit access to support programs. This advantage first required that she recognize her own blameworthiness for her life's circumstances. Stacey achieved this by disallowing herself to have the expectation for support. Paradoxically it was precisely her refraining from the expectation for support that helped Stacey to increase her support options. This paradox may be partially explained by American therapeutic models and treatment for addiction. In *Scripting Addiction* Carr (2011) explains that American addiction recovery programs endeavor to teach women how to reveal their inner thoughts and feelings vis-à-vis language unmediated by "denials" of personal culpability. In some cases, however, women "flip the script" (191), telling people what they want to hear as a means of resisting the therapeutic interaction and asserting their agency in a situation over which they may have little control. Read in this way, Stacey's discussion of her undeserving status can be seen in part as a speech performance through which she could communicate acceptance of personal responsibility for the conditions of her life. Stacey had then presumably seen the error of her ways and, by virtue of this knowledge of her own culpability, accepted that she was undeserving of support. Her acknowledgment of gratitude for the generosity of care providers reinforced her recognition of self-blame.

DeeDee, too, was a former illicit drug user who well understood the strategic usefulness of personal responsibility and thankfulness. At the initiation of this research, she had been sober for nearly five years. Following her discharge from the military and a two-year stint of incarceration for credit card fraud, DeeDee had "pulled it together." Although she lived with her mother and had few financial burdens, DeeDee often said that she was thankful Health Partnership existed, even if she did not usually need to access its financial or medical support services. In an interview she described this gratitude she felt: "Nobody has to help you. Ever. You can be out there on your own. I just try to be thankful that I can get whatever little bit I can. I may not need money from them, but I can come down here and get my little food and just be thankful for that."

Stable women's gratitude was often rooted in prior personal experiences of material want. It was true that without Health Partnership, they would have likely faced financial crises and burdens with no other options for help. By virtue of federal mandate, Ryan White programs were necessarily the last stop along the health and human services continuum. Yet stable women never openly critiqued weaknesses in the social safety system that led them to need access to services from *the* provider of last resort; instead, they consistently described their reasons for gratitude in the language and values of individualism. Thus, Stacey placed the onus of blame for her living conditions on herself while simultaneously positioning support services as a gift rather than an entitlement. DeeDee similarly acknowledged support services as a gift to which she was not entitled. In both cases the women emphasized their life circumstances as outcomes of individual decisions and actions rather than as outcomes of structural vulnerability.

Stable women further contrasted their feelings of gratitude in relation to the purported ingratitude of others. This strategy had the effect of reinforcing the stereotype that HIV/AIDS care clients were entitled, acting as though they were owed assistance, and otherwise socially inappropriate, or appearing ungrateful and not behaving deferentially. Later during our conversation about the recovery house, for example, Stacey made clear her own disdain for others' lack of appreciation: "I see some people that come around here, and they're cutting up, and they talk nasty and stuff. They feel like people owe them something. They don't say 'please' or 'thank you.' They just think that people there are there just to be serving them because they got HIV and they're mad."

Stacey communicated her social distance from "other" women, a strategy that was particularly meaningful in a context of diminishing HIV/AIDS resources. Dwindling financial and in-kind support options created competition among the women. Policies such as "first come, first served" coupled with the discretion that individual service providers wielded for determining programmatic services eligibility left many women feeling as though they had to prove their need and/or eligibility was greater than that of other applicants (Davis 2006). Thus it was not enough for stable women to model gratitude; they felt they also had to socially separate themselves from those clients presumed as undesirable. Social distance from the general client population quickly had become imperative in this competitive setting.

Stable women also exemplified personal values and service utilization habits commensurate with agency ideals concerning proper decorum and appropriate services use. To put it simply, stable women were well behaved in the sense that their lives were difficult to reconcile with popular stereotypes depicting impoverished Black women as hostile, promiscuous, and exploitative recipients of public resources (Collins 2001). Joan, for example, was diagnosed with HIV disease just after high school. At that time she canceled her enrollment in college courses and focused, instead, on caring for her health. She soon married her boyfriend, who was also HIV-positive. Together they sought to beat the odds and live well with HIV disease. Although living well below the poverty line at the time of this research, Joan and her husband rented a small two-bedroom home in a middle-class neighborhood. They gardened, practiced meditation, and enjoyed walking for fitness. They also negotiated heavily discounted memberships to the local YMCA and managed to afford an occasional date night at the movies. In small ways the two enjoyed amenities of a middle-class life. "Living well" for Joan meant "enjoying life by making time and a way to live right," which included caring for her health and maintaining good working relationships with her physicians and care providers. During a conversation about her health care strategies, Joan described why she had a good relationship with her HIV case manager: "Well, she saw the things that I was capable of doing. She saw the skills, the way I talked, um, me having a support group, my husband. The things we do, the resources we bring back to them—all of that. And that's when she opened up to me, and I opened up more to her."

Joan described that she and her case manager worked well together because the case manager found her to be compatible with personal and institutional ideals concerning marriage, empathy, and community involvement. She further explained her interpersonal appeal: "Well, me personally, I've seen clients complain about case management, and they don't realize how much of a big load case managers have, and they don't have patience—the clients don't. But they don't realize what they have to do."

Joan appreciated the busy schedules of case managers, and because she recognized how challenging their jobs were, she rarely complained of service-related difficulties. More important she explained this recognition in relation to a presumed client norm. The normative client was unaware of, or perhaps unimpressed with, the long hours many case managers work. Indeed, service providers often lamented that impatient clients lose sight of how much work may be involved with providing assistance for a person with chronic and multiple needs. Stable women, in contrast, empathized with care providers because they shared common social values whereas "challenging" clients were not presumed to do so.

Perhaps most important, stable women were personally responsible in ways that were compatible with agency directives and managed federal funds efficiently. Thus in contrast to irresponsible women, *they* could be trusted not to "abuse" services by using them in an "irresponsible" way. "Appropriate" service use was critical to agency survival. Care providers kept detailed records of their financial allocations and were expected to justify each dollar spent. In addition, as in other states, North Carolina and its HIV/AIDS-related agencies needed to spend all of the money allocated through the Ryan White CARE Act for a given fiscal year, or they would lose the amount of unspent funds the following fiscal year. At the same time, because Health Partnership employees billed Ryan White for services provided, the agency's bankroll covered its initial costs until the state HIV/AIDS consortium reimbursed them;

thus Health Partnership experienced lean periods in its funding cycle when money was in short supply. The agency ran out of money to extend approximately twice a year. During these periods, it had no choice but to wait for the distribution of Ryan White reimbursement funds before providing any more assistance. In 2008 it experienced a three-week suspension of emergency financial assistance. During that time it necessarily turned away several clients as there simply was no money available to help them. Clients were expected to understand these ebbs and flows of federal funding and adjust their service use accordingly.

Clients could potentially misuse services in several ways. The most common offense, however, was to display a service use pattern of "dependence." Women who seemed to consume resources consistently without trying to be self-sufficient were regarded as acting selfishly and wastefully. Thus they represented a threat to the financial survival of Health Partnership. Debdai, for example, was one stable woman for whom the stereotypes of dependence were particularly salient. As a longtime recipient of public aid and public health care benefits, Debdai drew sharp distinctions between herself and socially different women living under similar economic circumstances. Consider Debdai's explanation concerning why she believes she always received the support she requested: "They know who's doing right and who's not. If I came in every month, I could see. My record of not using the services is proof. Sometimes you have to look at the person and not by the book. But my no drug use speaks for itself. I don't take everything that's offered—just what I need. I don't even take everything they give me at the food pantry. I always give back what I can't use or I already have, but they continue to help those that aren't even trying."

Debdai equated drug addiction with "not trying" to comply with behavioral prescriptions concerning the community good and personal gratitude. Her habit of returning food pantry items that she could not use and avoiding requests for emergency assistance fell well within the boundaries of what agency staff considered as appropriate usage of Treatment Modernization Act resources. Care providers appreciated this type of discretionary service use because those resources could be distributed to someone who really needed them. A woman who accepted assistance with the intention of generating profit, of giving resources to an HIV-negative friend, or of throwing them away would have been considered as acting without regard for the greater good of the community and the financial sustainability of the organization. Building a history and reputation of socially appropriate service use thus provided one means by which stable women could strengthen their social capital and, in turn, their institutional networks. These networks wielded support even in times of financial stress among care programs.

For example, Charlotte needed rental assistance during a community-wide spending freeze on Ryan White emergency assistance funds. For close to three months service providers struggled to assist clients with their housing and health needs. New contracts concerning housing and rental assistance programs for the new fiscal year had not yet arrived in North Carolina; thus Ryan White funds simply were not yet available. Rather than see her evicted or potentially succumb to further financial crisis, Health Partnership employees relaxed the rules. The new Ryan White contracts and funds were already in place for the medical case management/treatment adherence program, so the agency temporarily diverted Charlotte's rent money from this account until it could be replaced by money earmarked specifically as emergency assistance dollars. In this way Charlotte's strategic use of services and good working relationship with care providers translated into a best possible outcome in a context of resource scarcity.

Finally stable women further proved their personal responsibility by fulfilling skills-based roles as support group organizers, Community Advisory Board members, public speakers, and designated role models and mentors for women who struggled with medication adherence and/ or addiction recovery. Their activities educated community members and the general public about the conditions of survival with HIV disease and, at the same time, helped to alleviate resource scarcity and/or personnel challenges. These women volunteered with children's literacy programs and church activities and/or continued to work in the professional and semiprofessional world.

DeeDee, for example, was a professional woman who continuously sought meaningful employment. In her spare time DeeDee volunteered for a children's literacy program at a nearby community center, where she read to young children who could not yet read and tutored older children who found reading difficult. At the beginning of this research, DeeDee came to Health Partnership weekly. She would stop by just to help out with food pantry duties and general office maintenance. I often talked with her as she vacuumed, cleaned bathrooms, or helped unload shipments of donated food. After a few months a program employee suggested that DeeDee take on a different type of volunteer role. Her excellent communication skills and her outgoing and jovial personality qualified her to act as a representative of sorts on behalf of the HIV-positive community. DeeDee soon began occasionally speaking at area high schools about HIV prevention. She reported that her sense of humor, respectable style of dress, and young looks rendered her an effective speaker to the youths. She viewed herself as someone with whom young women could relate. In an informal conversation she explained, "Those little girls, they just love me. They like, 'Oh Miss DeeDee, we want to be like you when we grow up. You so fun.' I love it, girl, because I love kids. And they see that, yeah, I got this, but I'm like Tyra Banks—'So what?'"

DeeDee enjoyed public speaking because she felt that her message reached a population that was often skeptical of adults. Her Tyra Banks "so what" attitude sent a message to youths who might otherwise stigmatize persons living with HIV disease. DeeDee took pride in her challenge to popular stereotypes concerning low-income women with HIV. She believed her humor, stylish clothing, positive attitude, and desire to own a home flew in the face of popular and racist images that she described as depicting poor women of color as "house-shoe wearing, scarf-around-the-head women." DeeDee's foray into the spotlight as a public speaker transformed her volunteer status into what can be considered as a "professional volunteer."

Professional volunteer work included activities requiring particular skills and organizational habits because it most often took place at the intersections between the HIV-positive community and the general public. Public speaking skills, knowledge of computers, and writing skills were the capabilities most often required of women who performed volunteer activities in public settings. Joan, for example, organized and led two support groups, including one group focused on the achievement of personal life goals. In between bimonthly meetings, Joan created computer-generated fliers and distributed them via email to different service organizations in Midway. She created meeting agendas and researched information concerning various clinical trials, educational forums, and resource opportunities in the area. Her work facilitated client investment in the many local HIV/AIDS-related venues.

The women's professional volunteer activities generated a variety of benefits. First, coordinating support groups, participating in CAB meetings, and public speaking put them into direct, informal contact with a variety of service providers. These occasions allowed care providers more opportunities to talk with the women about topics other than their financial needs or health concerns. For example, Joan often informed Monica about the various clinical trials taking place in Midway. The two would talk briefly about new medications on the horizon and conditions of eligibility for the study. Oftentimes these conversations unfolded into exchanges about the general challenges of counseling clients. Joan's status as a support group organizer lent her opinions and perspectives a kind of professional credibility non-volunteers tended to lack. Second, professional volunteer activities often indebted service providers to stable women in at least some small way. Stable women's agreement to speak at a public event or drum up participants for special programs helped agency employees meet grant requirements.

While volunteers discussed their work as personally satisfying and empowering, they also readily acknowledged that volunteerism fulfilled a perceived social obligation to Health Partnership. The dictates of personal responsibility required the women to "earn" (and thereby deserve) the support they received. To earn support was a moral as well as an economic endeavor. Organizing and running a support group provided one way to assist the agency with funding requests and justification. Joan's support group was a peer counseling effort that demonstrated to private donors in particular that agency programs worked, were community based, and were culturally appropriate. When the stable women organized or spoke at local events, they also freed providers to use their energy elsewhere to benefit the community and the agency. Donating their labor in this way precluded the women from being seen as dependent and entitled in a policy context that seeks to "liberate" the poor from welfare. Stable women thus had more than cultivated surrogate social networks; they had also defined community-specific terms of moral belonging by demonstrating personal responsibility and charitable giving.

Gratitude and moral uprightness, appropriate use of services, and skills-based volunteerism were part of what enabled stable women to occasionally utilize financial resources for what was legislatively considered as material wants rather than needs. Their material wants included items beyond food, shelter, clothing, and medical care. Although many women described living in conditions of relative comfort, they still lived their lives below the poverty line; thus the women who sought socioeconomic advancement needed programmatic services support to work for them in some nontraditional ways. Stable women tended to time their use of services for nontraditional needs to coincide with fiscal year "spend downs" and/or contract reimbursements; that is, their requests coincided with cash influxes.[2] That way stable women's requests were not likely to keep other clients, perhaps with more immediate needs, from receiving services. Instead, their use of services could be regarded as responsible in the sense that they were helping the organization spend their funds and ensure that the next fiscal year would include at least the same amount of federal funding.

Debdai, for example, used Ryan White spend-down resources to help her afford modest travel. She explained:

> I use these programs usually in the late spring or early summer because they allow me to do summer trips. You can think, like, if I can save like eighty or a hundred dollars a month, how a difference that makes. I can save some money for that because I go for assistance just like every two or three months. By that time, the bill has doubled so I can put all that money back. And then the bill comes after it's been settled, and I still have to pay that month's rent even though they've taken care of the other two or three months. But there's no jeopardy for two months, so you really end up getting four months leeway with your rent. You get more credit when you let the bill go.

Debdai's strategic use of emergency assistance services enabled her to save money for summer vacations. Over the years she found that "letting a bill go" essentially meant that she would receive that much more in assistance funds. Using Ryan White services as a last resort before eviction, rather than as a last resort for a single month, helped her to save more of her disability income. Debdai's rent was $82 per month, meaning that it would take her at least three or four months to save the money needed for a bus trip to visit family in New York. While some service providers viewed the trip home as a "nonessential" need, it was important to Debdai because it allowed her stay connected with family and friends. These social connections were an important part of Debdai's self-esteem and mental health. Maintaining these relationships meant that she had several individuals to whom she could turn in times of emotional distress.

Although stable women did not typically have disposable income for nonessential needs, such as car maintenance, vacations, and savings accounts, they improvised strategies for meeting those needs. Stable women operated in the context of a health care system that was partially based on ideas concerning the focus on adherence, the client-provider partnership, and the responsibility to volunteer. In this context displays of gratitude, appropriate uses of services, and professional volunteer activities enabled the women to personalize their relationships with service providers by highlighting the social similarities between them. In turn service providers could rely upon stable women to participate at community events and publicly demonstrate the efficacy of the programs they worked so hard to administer. Stable women were experts at negotiating access to support services precisely because they learned how to transform behavioral modification strategies into social capital. In the process they reconfigured an institutional terrain aimed at fiscal oversight and self-management into a surrogate social network.

Precariously Situated Women and Social Network Surrogacy

Precariously situated women also actively sought to build personal alliances with case managers, counselors, and other service program employees; however, they were less successful than their stable counterparts when it came to realizing social capital in this context. Daily life conditions of uncertainty and hardship for precariously situated women often challenged even their most earnest attempts to build relationships with care providers. Precariously situated women, though, were rarely met with overt judgment or harsh stereotypes by Health Partnership employees, for most service providers were acutely aware of the challenges the women faced and their sensitivities to historically driven imagery and negative stereotypes concerning poor women of color. Providers generally communicated respect and empathy to precariously situated women by committing their names to memory, asking about loved ones during informal conversations, and endeavoring to maintain accurate appointment schedules and client files. A general feeling of familiarity and conviviality permeated most client-provider relationships. A few socially popular precariously situated women, such as Lady E. and Lisa, enjoyed extra attention in the form of casual conversation, humorous quips, and friendly hugs. Overall, however, precariously situated women were less effective than their stable counterparts in transforming programmatic service interactions into functioning social networks. This was, in part, because federal policy and local services protocol were not designed to accommodate service needs and material realities associated with fluctuating life circumstances. As a result the women relied on unsanctioned, and usually self-destructive, strategies for stability.

Given persistent changes in housing, income, and social circumstances, precariously situated women reported making an average of four financial assistance requests each year, and those women who experienced a period of instability in their lives clearly sought more support.[3] Health Partnership employees carefully reviewed escalating appeals for support in relation to the women's substance abuse issues, personal life circumstances, and service use history. Care providers reviewed client files, spoke with colleagues administering psychosocial and substance abuse services, and consulted with the director of client services before promising financial support to a woman who had recently used the service. Despite steps taken toward proving their moral uprightness, the women in this group frequently failed to demonstrate their personal responsibility in an unequivocal way. Specifically care providers scrutinized the women in this group as "entitled." As explained in chapter 4, the term "entitlement" referred to a negatively valued attitude of being owed something.

Notions of entitlement were central to local definitions of how clients could potentially misuse programmatic services, and they arose, in part, because care providers generally interpreted the Treatment Modernization Act through the lens of neoliberal political rhetoric asserting that poor women have been improperly socialized to expect and depend on state-sponsored aid. The idea was that so-called entitled women used aid services simply (and wantonly) because they could. Precariously situated women, however, used the term "entitlement" in the sense of statutory rights conferred to a group. Women were entitled to receive services on the basis of their technical eligibility for services. Indeed, many precariously situated women who felt ignored, shortchanged, or unnecessarily excluded by programmatic service employees and procedures asserted their statutory entitlement to support.

Kareese was one woman who frequently asserted her technical entitlement to services as a service use strategy. She frequently requested support for monthly bills partially because her husband often failed to pay his half of their expenses. Her addiction to crack and alcohol also posed considerable financial burdens on their household. Given her known addiction and the frequency of her requests, providers periodically denied Kareese's applications for assistance. Following one such denial, she explained: "I ain't no stupid ass. . . . I know that they can't do nothing for me every month. I'm getting a check. But when you in a financial bind like me. . . . That should have helped us because of that. That's they job. The money is there to help me."

From Kareese's perspective, she had a *right* to use Ryan White emergency assistance funds. Her right was based on her biological status as HIV-positive and on her demonstrable need for cash assistance. In that sense, Kareese *was* technically entitled to support services. And reminding employees of her technical right was a strategy for self-preservation in a context where she felt she had been judged and perhaps mistakenly dismissed. "They just judge me like I don't deserve help because I be using crack sometimes," she explained. "The way I see it is that this money is supposed to help me because of that." Even so perhaps what Kareese failed to realize was that demonstrating her conformance with market-oriented social values had become imperative in this competitive setting. Her assertion of entitlement to HIV/AIDS-related support defined the terms under which her request was denied.

Providers' main strategy for dealing with entitled clients was thus to firmly deny any requests for support that were deemed inappropriate, lest they seem complicit with an improper use of funds. Muriel, for example, had long suffered financial hardship. In December 2007 she took a trip home to New York and returned to find that her house had been robbed. She lost everything, including the food in her cabinets, a television, appliances, and clothing. Muriel also dealt with a messy leak in her ceiling and a mice infestation in her apartment. She wanted to move into a nicer apartment in a safer neighborhood, but with only $546 per month, affording a new place to live was a difficult task. She was ineligible for down payment and/or first month's rental assistance because she was already housed. Providers could not guarantee that if she broke her lease and sought eviction, they would have the resources to help her reestablish a residence. Muriel thus devised a long-term strategy for increasing her monthly income by officially reestablishing residency in New York City while still informally living in Midway. She estimated that disability payments based on the cost of living in New York would exceed what was offered in Midway by at least an extra $200 each month. Muriel justified her plans by pointing out that she currently rented a storage locker in New York, so technically she participated in the state economy. She had only to compile the appropriate paperwork.

One afternoon Muriel came to Health Partnership with a lease for an apartment in New York City. A friend had mailed her a copy so that she could figure out how to make the lease appear as if it were in her own name. Borrowing correction fluid from the reception desk, she covered her friend's name as the lessee. Next she asked employees if they could help her type her name on the document. As it so happened, Natasha had an old typewriter in her office. Natasha, a licensed social worker, prepared the document for Muriel and asked, "What is it that I'm doing here?" Muriel vaguely responded that she needed a lease for her disability income claims. Natasha responded, "But this is a lease for New York, and you live in North Carolina. No, I'm not doing this. I won't lie to the federal government for you." Now visibly frustrated, Muriel retorted, "I'm not asking you to lie. I'm asking you to type this for me. That's it. You don't even know what's going on." Muriel then hastily left Health Partnership, angry that she had been so quickly denied the help she wanted. From Natasha's perspective, however, Muriel was committing welfare fraud, a charge potentially damaging to all involved. Muriel's support needs and requests were thus not open for discussion.

Precariously situated women generally had inconsistent relationships with care providers. In cases where women continuously struggled month after month to secure support and make ends meet, relations were strained. Kareese was one woman for whom the client-provider relationship was tricky. She frequently needed support as a result of her chemical dependency and her economic arrangements with her husband. Between the two of them, they requested financial assistance nearly every other month. Separate finances and separate social lives revolving around addiction usually meant that at least one of them was without some portion of her or his half of the rent. Care providers were never really sure whether Kareese and her husband sometimes "played the system" together; therefore, they often met her requests with skepticism. Strained relationships such as this one tended to remain institutional in nature, meaning that the women could not compel service providers to be flexible with program guidelines. Institutional relationships, in this sense, were characterized by a lack of power sharing between providers and clients that might result in personal favors, professional or semiprofessional opportunities, and/or increased access to Ryan White–related resources. Indeed, institutional relationships did not extend beyond the boundaries of what could be considered in this context as "typical" client-provider relationships. In these "typical" relationships, providers tended to strictly adhere to appointment scheduling guidelines and observe official service provision protocol.

Despite daily life challenges associated with financial instability, mental illness, and/or addiction, precariously situated women sometimes made considerable progress toward improving their daily life conditions in ways that were compatible with the values of personal responsibility embedded in the TMA and agency-sponsored programs. Lady E. was one temporarily stable woman who seemed well poised to achieve long-term stability. At the beginning of our research relationship, Lady E. had just taken dramatic steps toward "living right." Despite having zero income, a recent diagnosis with AIDS, and a serious heart condition, she was committed to "improving the self to improve [her] life." This goal meant she had to "wipe the slate clean," so to speak, and clear any outstanding debt and legal matters. She wanted to be as healthy as possible and so underwent a ninth angioplasty procedure to increase her chances for physical fitness. Following recovery from the procedure, Lady E. turned herself in to local authorities for outstanding arrest warrants. She served six months in jail before working with a local mental health agency to clear outstanding debts owed to landlords and utility companies.

Eight months into this research and approximately eighteen months after she began her life anew, Lady E. had made dramatic progress in her daily life conditions. First and foremost, her HIV lab work indicated that she was no longer in immediate danger for AIDS-related complications. With 400 CD4 cells and a viral load of only 1,200 replications, she was comfortable with her HIV status. Lady E. at this time rented a room in a boardinghouse. She felt the room was a step backward in one sense because it was small and she had to share a kitchen and bathroom with strangers. Conversely, she acknowledged that renting the room made good financial sense, for she had lived before in an apartment she could not afford. While she had zero income, Health Partnership, Social Services, and a local mental health agency had paid her rent, but now that her disability had been reinstated, she was expected to pay her own rent. She simply could not afford the apartment and pay her other bills. Moving into the affordable boardinghouse signified an important step toward her future plans of self-sufficiency.

In addition to securing an affordable room, Lady E. strategically used the disability back pay she received. Her strategy paid off when service providers recognized her as a responsible person. She explained, "When I got my lump sum, which was $1,700, I paid for a burial plan. I paid for a computer because I really wanted it even though I couldn't afford the Internet at first. I got a dining room set, and I got a decent mattress for my bed because my back was always killing me. I didn't waste it away. And what happened was the workers came and they seen. 'She didn't get high. She didn't waste that money. She's still going to group. This is where her money went.'"

Lady E.'s strategies for long-term financial stability and substance abuse recovery began to pay off in terms of access to financial resources. Staff saw her as a person who did not waste precious resources. She was newly positioned in the realm of HIV/AIDS services as a client who had taken on the personal responsibility to abstain from illicit drug use, attend to HIV-related health needs, and properly manage financial matters.

Lady E. next began taking steps toward receiving a small business license so that she could formally sell the beaded necklaces and bracelets she made "to keep her mind from [thinking about] drugs." She hoped to turn her small business into an Internet enterprise so that she could reach a wider population of potential buyers. She managed a small business loan and a business credit card. Lady E. prided herself on having that money and not spending it on drugs.

Lady E.'s hard-earned sobriety and relative stability opened doors that she never thought possible. Health Partnership staff began supporting her business by buying jewelry and paying her to fix old pieces in need of repair. At one point she estimated that she earned an extra $40 per week from agency staff alone. Some staff would refer friends to Lady E. so that they could shop her jewelry collection.

During this time, service providers relaxed the rules for Lady E.; she was now able to cancel and reschedule appointments, however late the notice, with no repercussions. In addition, the Comprehensive Risk Counseling and Services counselor felt comfortable enough to advance Lady E. the $15 Wal-Mart gift card she received for each CRCS session she attended. Paula, the CRCS counselor, knew that Lady E. looked forward to her monthly gift card so that she could buy new beads for her business. Lady E. always made up her appointments, so the advances were never perceived as a service delivery problem.

One month before I exited the field in 2008, however, Lady E. began experiencing small setbacks in her financial efforts. Gas prices soared, grocery prices rose, and Health Partnership employees began feeling the crunch of the looming economic recession. Casual conversation at the office tended to revolve around financial hardship and fear of agency cutbacks. Employees were no longer able to purchase Lady E.'s jewelry on a regular basis. She had come to rely on the extra $40 per week and was disappointed when that money was no longer an option. She conceded, however, that program employees owed her nothing. The relationships she was cultivating were not based on reciprocity. Lady E. provided employees with a valuable service when she repaired their jewelry and created custom pieces for them; however, because they paid her, this type of work did not create the conditions under which employees would become indebted to Lady E. in any way. Although nobody ever said as much, I had the impression that employees felt they were doing Lady E. a favor by supporting her fledgling business. They sometimes discussed "scrounging up old jewelry" in need of repair and buying necklaces they "didn't really need." Even as service providers appreciated Lady E.'s ingenuity and fine craftsmanship, the best option for personalizing her institutional networks would have been doing community volunteer work. Precariously situated women found it difficult, however, to break into the role most valued by service professionals—namely, that of the professional volunteer.

Precariously situated women did accomplish important tasks in their volunteer work, even if it was not generally considered as professional or skills based. As noted earlier, for example, Lisa fulfilled the role of outreach worker for a Health Partnership affiliate that implemented funds from Medicaid and the Centers for Disease Control and Prevention for HIV/AIDS case management and prevention programs. Her main task was to conduct street outreach about safer sex practices. She also recruited small groups of people to attend the "safer sex parties" that the affiliate hosted. For nearly ten years she donated her time and energy to the organization. In partial compensation for her work of recruiting otherwise disinclined groups to learn about safer sex, each month the organization gave her a $100 gift card to Wal-Mart.

One evening after a church service for the Black Church Week of Prayer, Lisa talked with a representative of the church's youth ministries about scheduling a safer sex party.[4] She explained that she performed volunteer work with a local HIV/AIDS service organization, and the representative invited Lisa to call her later in the week to talk further about the goal of the party. Later that week Lisa called me to tell me that she had achieved the "biggest coup ever": the church was willing to schedule an event outside the Black Church Week of Prayer. Lisa did not get to organize a church-friendly safer sex party, but she was able to arrange for the agency to provide an HIV/AIDS education and testing booth at the church's annual picnic.

On the Saturday morning of the picnic, I picked Lisa up at 9:00 a.m.

With a forty-ounce bottle of beer and a smile on her face, Lisa bounded out to the car. On the way to the event, she joked around that she should perhaps receive a prize of some sort for arranging an "AIDS event" on church property. Her face dropped when we arrived at the church. She did not see any of her fellow agency representatives. Church members bustled about, setting up tents, popcorn machines, stereo equipment, and games. After about ten minutes Lisa sat down on the sidewalk and started to cry. She lamented that "no matter what I do, they shit on me—just take it for granted that I'll come back." She reminded me that she had been overlooked at the Christmas party when other volunteers were recognized for their services. Lisa borrowed my cell phone to call the prevention program director. She cried harder when she learned that the service employees had changed their plans for the event without discussing them with her. When program employees did arrive more than an hour later, they failed to recognize Lisa's anger and frustration.

I believe, in part, their lack of recognition was due to Lisa's position. She was not a program administrator; therefore, she had little reason to assume she would be consulted about programmatic changes. I also believe they did not acknowledge Lisa's outburst as legitimate because of her apparent drunkenness. In any case Lisa was upset and unable to see the situation from the perspective of the organization's representatives. Lisa finally told them that she was "dropping them" and would no longer be a client at their organization. She later explained to me that her leaving was a form of punishment because they would not be able "to claim money from [her] Medicaid card anymore." One employee's response, however, summed up Lisa's conundrum: "You always say that, and you never do." She needed their services and support to make ends meet.

As Lisa's experience illuminates, some precariously situated women found breaking into professional volunteer activities and relationships socially and technically difficult. In some ways it was the result of being excluded from important decision-making processes, and in other ways it was the result of personal choices the women made concerning their communication strategies. In other cases addiction and/or depression made it hard for women to follow through or to be taken seriously as potential contributors to long-term or intensive tasks and activities. Still other women felt that the volunteer duties requested of them were degrading. Lady E., for example, was once asked to wear a sandwich board at a fund-raiser for a substance abuse program affiliated with but independent of Health Partnership. At the time she was a beneficiary of the program's ongoing financial support grant, which was coadministered by Health Partnership. Lady E. described her feelings about being asked to engage in this type of volunteerism: "You want me to stand up and hold a sign? And my treatment is already paid? Maybe I should have tried to hold the sign, but I felt like I'm not panhandling. I didn't panhandle for crack. You know I sure didn't panhandle for that, and I won't do it for this. . . . It's like I been getting high twenty-five years of my life. I have less because of it. I'm not less."

Despite the women's reservations concerning volunteer work, providers continued to prompt them into doing service activities. Some care providers viewed volunteer work as a source of self-esteem, which they otherwise presumed was lacking (see Goldstein 2001). Other care providers saw it as an informal condition of receiving services. This perception arose, in part, because volunteerism could fulfill the dictates of behavioral change and personal responsibility as it engaged the women in emotionally and/or fiscally productive work. Few precariously situated women volunteered their time in more formal ways; instead, they performed sporadic manual labor at Health Partnership, often coinciding with their personal appointment schedules. Care providers noticed and appreciated their work, but it did not satisfy what they saw as the women's responsibility for community survival and behavior change because it did not benefit the fiscal health of the organization. One case manager so described the lack of professional volunteerism among "entitled" clients: "If I help you, will you come help me get more money when we go speak at the capital? 'Well, no, I just can't deal with that. I can't deal with saying the words [HIV/AIDS].' But still you have no problem coming through the front door, not caring who's in the community, when you have to get your rent paid. Some just think they are entitled to money because of a disease but not responsible to take on the entitlement for advocacy."

In general precariously situated women struggled to demonstrate conformity with agency values and social mores. Daily life's uncertainties associated with addiction, financial insecurity, and material want shaped their service use strategies and relationships with care providers in contradictory ways; while they met the technical criteria for services use, they found personal responsibility difficult to convey. Precariously situated women experienced frequent negative interactions with care providers, even as they may have previously experienced successful applications for support. Their social relationships with care providers thus remained institutional and contingent on the nature of each specific support request.

Vulnerable Women and Social Network Surrogacy

In contrast to their more stable counterparts, vulnerable women struggled to no avail with creating and sustaining surrogate social networks. As highlighted in chapter 2, vulnerable women wrestled with meeting and maintaining the eligibility criteria for state-funded and federally funded antipoverty programs because of challenges associated with documenting their needs. For the same reasons, they seldom qualified for Health Partnership programs, even though the agency served as a provider of last resort. Their ineligibility was problematic for the women because it hindered relationship building with care providers. Disqualification for cash assistance services meant that the women had fewer opportunities for sharing the personal life stories and information that sometimes created bonds between providers of care and Health Partnership clients. In brief they were unable to endear themselves to care providers and thus remained undifferentiated from the general client population. Disqualification also meant fewer opportunities for vulnerable women to exhibit personal responsibility through appropriate service use. In addition chemical dependency, mental illness, and chronic homelessness impeded their abilities to draw on personal responsibility as a cultural resource. They were discredited and stigmatized further by virtue of their assumed indifference to the moral economy of HIV/AIDS care.

In the absence of formal channels for garnering support, vulnerable women relied on the empathy of service providers who cared about women's health and well-being. For example, Jamie was a woman with zero income who survived by living with her boyfriend and utilizing several food pantries. She was therefore technically homeless and absolutely impoverished. To complicate matters, Jamie suffered chronic diarrhea, a condition that left her unable to leave home for long periods and required extra money for laundry and disposable undergarments. Her primary source of assistance was her partner, who was also an HIV-positive individual living well below the federal poverty threshold. Because the lease and utility bills were in her partner's name, Jamie was unable to apply for financial assistance. On a few occasions, her partner requested support, but he failed to complete the appropriate paperwork. The two faced, more than once, eviction proceedings. During spend-down periods, Jamie had successfully lobbied for extra help and joint financial assistance appointments with her partner; however, her addiction to crack compromised her ability to negotiate with service professionals during spending freezes or lean periods in the funding cycle. When care providers were cautious of Jamie's requests for support, she resorted to using her AIDS diagnosis to persuade them to help her. She explained, "You have to roll out your symptoms and your sad story to get help at most of these places. Here you already know that I'm HIV-positive, so you know why the help is so important and what it means. But, you know, they can't always do it. They got their rules too. So I have to say all that about the diarrhea and tell my AIDS story again. And if I misused the funds I have with 'extracurricular activities,' then I may have to kind of like explain myself and tell the story again."

Jamie thus discussed how appealing to the providers' sense of compassion could alleviate technical disentitlement from many cash assistance services. This strategy sometimes worked precisely because Health Partnership employees generally cared about their clients' well-being. Most care providers wanted to prevent and/or alleviate any suffering that a client might experience. Jamie's tactic worked, however, only when employees had ample resources at their disposal. During agency-wide spend downs or when given a donated sum of money, employees could stretch the rules for an unsanctioned need such as disposable diapers or cash assistance for an otherwise "undeserving," or technically ineligible, client.

Given their technical ineligibility for Ryan White–funded services, most vulnerable women relied on Medicaid case management as their primary source of health-related support. In relation to Health Partnership's programs, Medicaid case management was designed as a point of access and care retention. Medicaid case managers requested support on behalf of the women, verified their eligibility for services, and assisted with their procedural compliance. Despite community-wide consumerist rhetoric of HIV/AIDS care, the women in this group mostly experienced Medicaid case management as a continuation of their disfranchisement from TMA resources.

Nine out of eleven vulnerable women described scenarios where case managers billed Medicaid for services not provided. I frequently heard the women describe how they gave a new case manager a copy of their Medicaid card for billing purposes only to find that their case managers thereafter stayed out of reach until it was time to conduct an annual update. Health Partnership was attuned to these issues but could do little to dissuade predatory Medicaid case managers. Health Partnership entertained the idea of contracting with Medicaid but, to my knowledge, never cultivated the program.

Sharon was one woman for whom Medicaid services proved unreliable. She lived with her brother and sister-in-law in a one-bedroom house and was enrolled in substance abuse programs, but she had yet to receive treatment for the depression she faced. In her estimation her life could "get back on track if [she] had a place of [her] own." Sharon sought a case manager so that she could quickly find an affordable apartment in a relatively drug-free neighborhood; however, according to Sharon, her case manager avoided her phone calls and impromptu office visits. "I been calling my case manager, and I don't hear nothing. She say I got to take my Social Security and turn it over to them and let it be in their name. Well, I'm willing to do that if they hurry up and give me a place to stay. I'm just beat. I don't get no rest with where I'm staying."

As Sharon explained, her case manager refused to work with her until she formally designated her case management agency as her payee. Health Partnership employees sometimes questioned and criticized the payee role that some case management agencies took. Rumors circulated among Health Partnership clients and staff that some payees pooled their clients' disability checks instead of keeping separate accounts. This practice potentially meant that some clients did not always receive all of their cash benefits. Sharon was so uncomfortable living with her brother, though, that she considered relinquishing her monthly check to her case manager despite these accusations.

Other women in this group also explained that when they did meet with Medicaid case managers, it was unfruitful. The women requested that their case managers provide them with technical and emotional support while they tried to enroll in Ryan White–funded and other such social service programs. These requests were well within the purview of case management programming, and, in fact, case managers sometimes described their jobs in similar terms. As Jonathon, a Medicaid case manager who spoke at a community event, put it, "We provide people with financial and technical assistance. We don't do it for you, but we show you how. We can walk you through the system and give you that emotional piece that you might need to feel supported and be successful." Contrary to these supportive intentions, vulnerable women viewed their relationships with Medicaid case managers as unhelpful and sometimes demeaning. Vulnerable women felt as though their requests were disregarded when Medicaid case managers referred them to Health Partnership. Tasha lamented, "They [Medicaid case managers] ain't worth no two damn cents because they send us over here [Health Partnership]. And we came here first, you know. They send you somewhere you already been turned down at, know what I mean? You got all those people working there, and the most thing I can get out of there is a couple of bags of food."

Tasha explained that her Medicaid case manager provided her with referrals rather than actually assisting with support requests. She questioned the point of having a case manager if that person could not physically assist the women in gaining access services. Physical assistance was especially important for women such as Tasha who experienced chronic and multiple barriers to care as a result of addiction, mental illness, and/or legal issues.

Similarly Chantelle had long since stopped trying to work with case managers whom she perceived as unconcerned with clients who were relatively poor in relation to other clients. In Chantelle's estimation her experiences as a chronically homeless woman with no means of income and a long-term addiction to crack and alcohol translated into social devaluation.

> Well, how about this here? I was asking my case manager for help getting me housing, finding a job, helping me stay clean. I got a termination letter from the Social Security place—from disability. I didn't understand what it meant, and I went to my case manager's office. I said, "Excuse me, I need to see you." She said, "Later, Chantelle. I'm too busy for you right now." And you know what, five years and you haven't got me housing, you haven't got me a job, I haven't gotten any money. What are you doing for me? Seemed like you basically helping the people that got money. I'm the one that don't have. Help me, okay?

Chantelle's case manager told her that she did not "have time" for her at that point. Chantelle later recalled that remark as the pivotal moment that determined the dissolution of their client-provider relationship. She felt that particular response was more or less reflective of the dynamics that had taken place for five years. Chantelle had recertified every year with her case manager, regularly requested assistance, and used the food pantry at the Medicaid case management agency; however, she was still not positioned to be considered as a service priority because she lacked a lease and utility bills in her name. Thus the services she could receive were limited. Until she achieved sobriety and could document her residency or ability to pay rent, a case manager could not do much for her in the way of financial support.

Rosalind encountered a similar experience when she signed up for Medicaid case management. She more generally lamented, "I quit her, and now I'm my own case manager. What do I need you for? For you to work my Medicaid card? You know but they do bring by food and then they write out plans and stuff for you, but those plans stay that way— just written down."

In Rosalind's estimation Medicaid case managers function to "work" the women's Medicaid cards, meaning case managers bill Medicaid for services not provided. Many women, regardless of their social and economic positions within the broader system of HIV/AIDS care and support services, were skeptical of case managers. Vulnerable women felt this potential dynamic acutely in the context of their own suffering. As a further insult to their senses of justice and fairness, Health Partnership clients sometimes admired their case managers' nice cars and fancy clothes. Tasha mused aloud that "my Medicaid card probably bought that nice little shirt."

In this context the vulnerable women's relationships to Health Partnership were situational and, in the end, financially unsustainable. Vulnerable women were sometimes able to garner support through programmatic services during times when donor-driven resources were relatively plentiful. That support, however, often stopped short of truly meeting vulnerable women's needs because they were far more intensive than what periodic and program-specific donations could cover.

Vulnerable women sometimes received support when challenging circumstances proved beyond their control. In the months before I met Georgia, for example, she lived in an apartment, but she and her partner were evicted for nonpayment of rent. Social Services pledged to help Georgia secure the deposit for another place to stay. In the meantime, she and her partner rented a room for $400 per month in a boardinghouse. A few weeks into their stay at the boardinghouse, fellow tenants robbed the house of the stove, refrigerator, and furniture. The heat was turned off for failure of payment, a responsibility shirked by her landlord. Realizing that the winter months would bring cold weather, Georgia and her partner accepted partial assistance from Social Services and moved into a new apartment. At the same time, however, Georgia lost her ssdi income because the program revoked her eligibility for not reporting the small income she earned while she was briefly employed as a hotel maid.

Georgia turned to Health Partnership for further support. Together with Social Services, they paid her rent for three months while her partner paid the utility bills. Yet Georgia's financial situation did not improve over the three months she was able to receive emergency financial assistance. She and her partner tried to earn extra money by selling items found in the trash and in abandoned homes. The little money they earned from that, she explained, they sometimes used to buy crack. Health Partnership employees were aware of Georgia's chemical dependency issues. Indeed, Health Partnership was one place where women could candidly discuss their struggles without fear of legal repercussions. Georgia's substance abuse issues, however, meant that service providers closely monitored her money management. Although she had not yet been reinstated in the SSDI program, Georgia was cut off from emergency assistance funds until she demonstrated progress in substance abuse recovery or income-earning strategies. Case managers had to prove that assistance resulted in their clients' increased capacities for self-care and financial stability by demonstrating changes in their living conditions and service request patterns. Such proof justified the organization's spending and budget request for the next fiscal year. Georgia's experiences exemplified how Health Partnership employees guarded against their clients' inappropriate use of services that "enabled" them to use drugs. In turn, Health Partnership's strategies amplified the federal policy and local service dynamics through which vulnerable women negotiated requests for assistance.

In addition fellow clients who were well positioned within the care continuum quickly "put in their place" those vulnerable women who were perceived as ungrateful, irresponsible, or inappropriate. Elizabeth's experiences provide one example of how some women could be treated as an other given suboptimal daily life conditions. When I met Elizabeth, she had been recently released from jail for assault charges. As we talked Elizabeth sat across from me with her hands folded in her lap and a mild smile across her lips. She was calm, despite the stressful situation, as we discussed her living conditions. Upon her release from jail, Elizabeth learned that her husband had moved into a new rental home without telling her. She went to their old address and found him gone along with her clothing, furniture, and personal items. He did not call, visit, or write while she was incarcerated. She began asking neighbors, friends, and relatives if anyone knew where he had relocated. Finally a family member gave her the new address. Elizabeth went to the house and "reclaimed [her] place in [the] family." She reported that her husband was surprised to see her, but he did not resist her moving into the new home with him. Though she felt "a little embarrassed" that he would move without telling her, she was determined to stay positive about the situation. After all, she said, "he's my provider. He pays our bills and makes sure we got food to eat."

A few months after our initial interview, it appeared to me that Elizabeth began publicly displaying her frustration. Her husband was working only sporadically, and they had trouble affording the rent and utility bills. Elizabeth tried to volunteer at the food pantry as a means of gaining increased access to food, but the nutritionist quickly shut down her strategy because it was unfair to other clients who did not or could not volunteer. Elizabeth's uncharacteristic outrage prompted employees to wonder if her behavior meant that she had begun smoking crack again. They reiterated this idea one afternoon when she grabbed a donated purse from Raquel, another programmatic service participant. Elizabeth exclaimed that she had "wanted [the purse] from when it came in last week." Elizabeth dared Raquel to take it back from her. When Raquel declined to fight, Elizabeth began to yell that she hated one of the Health Partnership employees, referring to the employee as "a conniving bitch who thinks she rules the world." Elizabeth warned other clients not to trust her before being escorted from the building.

Soon after this incident, Elizabeth was banned from receiving services at Health Partnership. DeeDee, a model client, told the director of client services that she had witnessed Elizabeth stealing a large number of bus tickets from the agency's hiding spot. DeeDee herself had been painfully accused of stealing from Health Partnership long ago. She had also related to me that she hated "Elizabeth because she [is] an uppity bitch." Without any formal grievance process, Elizabeth lost her privileges at Health Partnership. She could not request assistance or access the food pantry for six months. In this case Elizabeth's disregard for agency-sanctioned strategies of communication and service use provided the means through which she could be further disenfranchised from federally funded HIV/AIDS health services.

Overall vulnerable women's inabilities to use institutional ties as a surrogate social network emerged from federal policies that did not reflect the social dynamics of physical vulnerability or the financial dynamics involved with addiction and incarceration. Because policy did not recognize variations in the conditions of poverty, service providers found it difficult to attend to vulnerable women's needs without "bending the rules" and thus endangering Health Partnership's relationship with state and federal funding sources. Federal policy guidelines instead favored women who were better positioned to display normative middle-class values and behaviors. Such a dynamic meant that African American women living with HIV disease in Midway experienced differential access to HIV-related services and programs designed to distribute material goods and cash assistance.

6. Using "Survival" to Survive, Part II

> You have to take responsibility because it's your life. If you don't take
> responsibility for your life with HIV and AIDS, honey, you going to lose
> something—your life. You go right on down if you don't stop sitting
> around doing all that drinking and smoking crack. . . . Nobody going
> to take care of you if you don't take care of yourself. Nobody. *You* get
> up and brush your damn hair. *You* take a shower. And *you* decide to do
> what that doctor tells you to do.
>
> RENE, an HIV-positive woman

In chapter 5 I describe performance of gratitude, moral uprightness, and
personal responsibility as behavior change goals that are differentially
realized among the women in this study. These strategies of self-
management, however, represent but one part of "survival" in its per-
formative sense. While self-management may be seen as a way to
decrease social spending on so-called undeserving populations, it also
may be seen as in the service of the public health mandate to use Ryan
White funds for the "greatest possible impact." Since the advent of highly
active antiretroviral therapy in 1996, the term "greatest possible impact"
has referred to the provision of medical treatment and testing. Thus the
most advantageously positioned women in this study also realized their
personal responsibility for health by becoming compliant and conversant
with a biomedical perspective on survival with HIV disease.

As with behavior change goals, the biomedical initiatives embedded
in survival discourse were also fashioned into eligibility criteria related
to oversight measures. For example, when I began this research in 2007,
the paperwork trail for eligibility in Ryan White programmatic services
in the post-TMA era had just begun. Prospective clients needed to sup-

ply Health Partnership with some form of identification, annual update or initial intake paperwork, proof of income, proof of insurance (if applicable), and up-to-date HIV blood work. With further implementation of the TMA throughout 2008, paperwork requirements had grown to include more specific documentation of need for oversight purposes. At that point a prospective client needed to complete the initial 2007 paperwork in addition to providing Health Partnership with a housing lease or bills in the applicant's name and documentation for assistance requests from three other agencies. Together these requirements presumably ensured that Ryan White funding was truly used as a provider of last resort.

When I returned to the field in 2009, North Carolina legislators had added yet another layer of paperwork requirements for ancillary services eligibility. New criteria emphasized compliance with medical treatment directives. Federally defined compliance was tracked via a series of laboratory diagnostics, including the initial two CD4 cell/HIV viral load counts taken three months apart within a twelve-month period. Locally, however, compliance also included proof of hepatitis B and C test results since the time of HIV diagnosis, proof of an annual syphilis test, and proof of an annual Pap smear. It was clear that Health Partnership was in the midst of scaling up the biomedical dimension of its therapeutic mission. The intention, as Jeremy explained, was both preemptive and "good": "It was one of those well-thought-out great ideas on paper, but when you go to carry it out, the paper starts cutting you. It was, 'We should provide more comprehensive, better care, and medicalize it so that the client gets more than just HIV treatment.' This is the direction of funding. If you look at it, medicalizing is the way to go. But we don't have enough money to carry it out right now, so instead of a benefit, it's a barrier. We are having to turn people away because they don't have all these test results."

Jeremy explained that viewing HIV/AIDS as a medical rather than as a social problem could have strategic value for people living with HIV/AIDS insofar as it provided a way to justify increased state support for health care services. Yet despite "growing pains," proverbial paper cuts, and systematic barriers to care under this increasingly medicalized version of U.S. HIV/AIDS care, the effects of prioritizing medical treatment programs have been primarily discussed in relation to resource-poor settings in underdeveloped and developing countries and perhaps rightfully so (see, for example, Koenig, Leondre, and Farmer 2004; Stover et al. 2006). After all the most recent and rapid expansion of HIV/AIDS care has been in the developing world and with great effect. According to UNAIDS and the World Health Organization (2006, 5), since 2002, a greatly expanded provision of antiretroviral treatment has led to an estimated two million life years gained in low- and middle-income countries. The elaboration of local health care infrastructure and expanded access to treatment and care have indeed produced promising results. But what of vulnerable populations living with HIV disease in developed countries? What impact has expansions to HIV-related medical care programming had for them? Here I bring U.S. HIV/AIDS care into the global public health conversation concerning scaled-up HIV/AIDS medical care as a way to shed light on benefits and unintended consequences of emphasizing medical treatment at the expense of social support programs.

In this chapter I consider in fine detail the scaling up of biomedicine within Midway's Ryan White system of care. I focus specifically on the women's varied experiences with the blood-work mandate, a programmatic service eligibility imperative that made obligatory the integration of laboratory diagnostics into one's routines of life and sense of survival. Building on insights concerning personal responsibility and deservingness in chapter 5, I frame the women's experiences with the blood-work mandate using the notion of biosocial inclusion as explained in chapter 4. By "biosocial inclusion" I am referring to how the women's statuses as HIV-positive granted them increased access to state resources. In other words, the women's diseased biology qualified them for social welfare programs that are not available to poor and HIV-negative women. To actually realize their technical qualification for state support, however, HIV-positive women had to continuously and willingly submit themselves to state-administered medical surveillance and associated perspectives on HIV health. In light of this requirement, I spotlight ways in which study participants variably used HIV-related blood work to make sense of their bodies and health, illuminating how techniques of medical surveillance articulated with social and material conditions of life in uneven ways.

Stable Women, Blood Work,
and Perceptions of HIV Disease

Stable women's participation in support groups, community events, and surrogate social networks gave them ample opportunities for discussing the biomedical facts of HIV disease and for learning treatment strategies and medical knowledge sanctioned by Health Partnership employees. Care providers and community educators felt it was important that women understood basic HIV-related medical knowledge. Collective educational events and meetings with support service providers and physicians provided venues for learning why CD4 cell counts and viral loads were regularly assessed measurements of health. The idea was that if women understood these basic medical principles, they could, as Monica put it, "see the medications working for them or their lack of adherence to the meds [might end up] killing them." In addition Health Partnership employees individually counseled the women to view themselves as "more than this disease" (Natasha) or as "in control of their health" (Monica). This messaging had the effect of prompting women to imagine laboratory blood work as a kind of "report card" telling them when they could move forward and regain or create a healthy lifestyle presumably founded on a realized commitment to medical treatment for HIV disease.

Stable women were highly conversant with this perspective. When asked to discuss how HIV affected their lives, they typically explained how they began to move forward with HIV disease by considering their disease course in relation to other chronic stresses and over time. This approach had the effect of positioning HIV as a less important concern than other life circumstances. Though most of the stable women in this study mentioned at some point that they would rather live without HIV infection, all things considered they felt as though it did not pose too big of a burden on their lives. Tamara, for example, described that she perceived HIV disease as less cumbersome than other chronic illnesses: "I realize that is not—from all the groups that I've been to and all the support groups, I've learned that even if I didn't have HIV, nobody knows when you're going to die. Because the medication, you know—the disease is treatable. And HIV is less worse than diabetes, cancer, hepatitis."

Tamara explained that HIV disease occupies a marginal place in the physicality of her daily life. Focusing attention on more immediate illnesses helped stable women to reframe HIV disease as a chronic health condition posing no insurmountable barriers to health and independence. Were it not for the actual ingestion of medicine, the women explained that they could live through an entire day, week, or year without "feeling HIV-positive"; that is, they perceived themselves as managing the disease and its symptoms so well that HIV was not an alarming presence in their lives. To this end, Debdai specifically explained, "The most thing that bothers me the most is my wear-and-tear arthritis, because that has hindered me more than my HIV. My HIV hasn't hindered me—that's the least of my worries. I've already rearranged my life to that style. It really doesn't bother me no more. I know I'll be around."

Stacey and Joan similarly described HIV disease as less burdensome than other chronic health concerns. As Stacey said, "I mean, this [HIV] is something to take care of. I mean, it's not something that you need to be messing with. But my real problem is that my legs ache all the time. [Doctors] don't know where it comes from. Ever since I had that blood clot, that's been my big health concern, really." And Joan explained, "My HIV is good, you know. For me, I know I really need to focus on the weight because my provider has told me that I need to make sure I exercise so I won't develop anything else, especially diabetes. Because of being overweight, you're more at risk of heart disease, high cholesterol—all of that."

Grace, meanwhile, described financial, rather than health-related, concerns as her most stressful life circumstance: "I never was afraid [of HIV]. I had friends living with it already when I found out. . . . What bothers me is that I want to be a whole person and work—'under the table,' as they call it. Disability just take care of your necessities—your basic bills, that's all. There's no more money left for nothing."

As Grace's explanation attests, stable women tended to perceive HIV infection in relative terms. The sense of calm they described, however, was acknowledged as an end point on a spectrum of stages for coming to terms with the disease. "Coming to terms" referred to their adoption of skills and knowledge related to anxiety management, medication adherence, and fluency in the language of diagnostic testing. For example, stable women all described early experiences of "feeling [HIV]-positive," meaning they felt anxiety and emotional distress in relation to their diagnoses. They contrasted these experiences with their current understandings of HIV disease as a lesser concern in their lives. For Joan, "that's where the therapy comes in. You have to learn to re-live. . . . It's hard, but you find the right mind frame to put this [HIV infection] in." Debdai also felt that with the help of her support group, she had made it through the process of coming to terms with the viral infection by learning to put HIV disease in proper perspective. "I started out with this outlook from my support group. They gave me a lot of help. I don't think I might not have made it. They helped me to recognize my depression and my feelings about HIV. They showed me that I was not alone and that I was not going to die. They also taught me that I can have personal successes if I keep working to it."

For other stable women, such as Tamara, they overcame their initial emotional distress by taking responsibility for medication adherence:

I—most of the time, I go about life like I don't have it. I don't dwell. I mean, I think like I have HIV or AIDS—whatever you want to call it. And I'm like, "Oh my God, I have the most—I have the monster." But I'm saying, "You know what? That monster is not bothering me, and I'm not bothering it." I have little army men inside of me. They are fighting this monster, and this monster is hiding from all of the little army men that are in there. This is a battle. . . . They need canons. It's like a parachute drop. They need their grenades. They need their bullets so I take the medicine, and there you go. It's empowering to know I provide them with what they need.

Tamara explained a by-now ubiquitous concept inculcated through the intersections among American commerce and the health care system (Martin 1994; Sontag 1990): health can be achieved through "training" and "arming" the immune system for "battle." The time she was able to devote to building a surrogate social network of HIV support service professionals and experienced peers paid off in terms of helping Tamara to reconceptualize HIV disease as a condition over which she had control. Her personal responsibility in this context was to make sure that her "little army men" had the ammunition they needed to succeed in battle.

Yet even as stable women steadily participated in health care regimens, they were critical of the meaning of blood work in their lives. Consider, for example, how Tamara explained her most recent laboratory results at the time of our second formal interview:

I can give blood this morning and then go back later on today, and they'll never be the same. They mean something, but it's not really nothing to stress out about. It's not exact. If I'm undetectable, it means that there's very little copies of the virus in my body. But then again, when I got diagnosed, you had to be over 400 or 300 and under to be undetectable. Every year they make it different. So even if it [the number of viral copies in the body] went up a little bit—say to 175, at one time that was undetectable. So why am I stressing? I was undetectable one time because I was under 175. You just can't hang on to the numbers too tight because they change.

Ashley and Stacey similarly explained that they asked their doctors to stop reporting the absolute numbers to them altogether. Ashley noted, "I said, 'Just tell me if my viral load goes way up or my CD4 is way down.' I don't want to know every number they take for me. I get too worried about nothing, and every little change don't really count. One thing I learned is that you got to look at the whole picture, not just one test." Stacey remarked, "I'm say[ing], 'Just tell me the direction'—if the numbers go up or down or stay the same. You just start worrying over numbers that by they self don't mean everything you need to know."

Stable women understood laboratory work as imperfect, incomplete, and situational. It led them to think of HIV disease in terms other than CD4 cell counts and viral loads. While their senses of well-being were bolstered by HIV blood work insofar as it indicated progress toward viral suppression, stable women heeded the advice of care providers to question the viability of single viral load testing results because the tests performed differently given such factors as time of day, stress levels, laboratory protocol, and technological developments over time (Corbett 2009). Stable women instead focused on managing their emotional sensitivity to the disease. This approach enabled them to control some aspect of their health experience while simultaneously diverting their attention from test results that were popularly known to fluctuate. With this in mind many stable women estimated that the realities of HIV infection and health could not be quantified, although favorable blood work played an important role in fostering their senses of a long-term future.

For this reason stable women discussed their experiences of HIV disease in terms of an emotional journey through which they gained acceptance of their medical status as HIV-positive. The journey, as they described, began with denial, fear, and, in some cases, anger or regret. Their subsequent emotional education and sophisticated understanding of the biomedical value of blood work enabled them to attend to future goals of stability. They had become, in effect, "therapeutic citizens," or individuals who were successful in appropriating meanings and practices of HIV blood work to bolster their claims for social membership, material resources, and the right to determine a future for themselves (see Nguyen et al. 2007). They were, as Charlotte put it, "survivors [who] came out the other side to use it all to an advantage." Indeed, they were survivors in the official senses of the term. Their HIV disease had become but one part of their lives well lived.

Precariously Situated Women, Blood Work, and Perceptions of HIV Disease

Some precariously situated women also experienced HIV disease and care as newfound means for changing their perceptions about life. After years of consideration and soul searching, a few precariously situated women came to regard HIV infection as a catalyst for conceiving of many life changes that were planned, if not made, since their diagnoses. Precariously situated women who experienced HIV disease as a catalyst for planning new and desirable life adventures had made self-defined progress in their attempts to improve their living conditions, health, and social circumstances. Lady E. explained her changing perceptions about living with HIV disease in this way: "I have less materialistic [sic]. I smoked up the mansion, the five-car garage, the Lex, the Benz. Believe me, I have. It got to do with who you are and your purpose for being here. And I have to let them know, 'Yeah, twenty-five years of addiction. Yeah, I got full-blown AIDS.' So what? I'm applying for Section 8. That's what I have collected in fifty years of living. That's not who I am. I am still good as gold, and I know it."

Lady E. spent twenty-five years of her life in the throes of crack addiction. Her past played an important part in shaping her outlook on HIV disease; it was the backdrop against which she measured her health progress. Yet she, like other precariously situated women, endured living conditions not always amenable to "going the distance" and realizing full personal responsibility for health. Her understanding of HIV disease reflected the daily challenges she faced in that it focused on immediate questions of life and death rather than on plans for an independent future. When asked to describe the effects of HIV on her daily life, she concentrated on how regularly attending an HIV-specific support group quelled persistent fears of imminent death and nihilism:

> I began to [feel] better after talking through it. And it [group therapy] got to be a group for people with HIV because you can't go into any old support group for addiction and be talking about "I got AIDS, I got Hep C." . . . People are like, "You so fucked up anyway, what the hell? Go ahead and die of AIDS." . . . I used to have a motto where I would tell somebody after I found out I was positive: "I got one foot in the grave, and the other one in quicksand. Come, go with me." . . . I don't say that now. And that's what a group will do for your mental [state].

Lady E. explained that her perspective on HIV disease changed over time. With the help of support group members and counselors, the virus no longer represented certain death. Moreover, it had become one turning point in a longer history of addiction, despair, and hard-earned progress. She had reconciled her past and remained firmly committed to the present as she learned to internalize messages of behavior change and medical compliance encoded in survival discourse. HIV, though not the lesser concern it was for stable women, was an illness made manageable by precariously situated women who learned to attend to its mental aspect.

Lady E. further explained that a healthy mental attitude was nurtured by her knowledge of HIV blood work. Given the health progress she had made, she believed that "there's comfort in that [laboratory work]. There's comfort in seeing that science work for you. You know? That's the real comfort. . . . Make them labs look good." Other precariously situated women, such as Kareese, also found comfort in "the numbers."

She explained, "So long as you know enough to know when you doing okay as far as, like, those numbers go, then you going to be fine emotionally." Contrary to the beliefs of stable women, and perhaps because precariously situated women had difficulty sustaining daily life stability, precariously situated women felt that paying close attention to the specific numbers reported in laboratory results provided a means for managing their mental stress. In daily life awash with uncertainty, laboratory analysis provided tangibility and direction for discerning one's success in the recovery or maintenance of health.

This careful attention to blood-work results further shaped the precariously situated women's explanations of their disease experience. They described HIV disease in terms of T cells, viral loads, and physical effects of infection. Even women who had not recently suffered or perceived any physical symptoms or side effects of HIV infection or medication explained life in physical terms. Treva, for example, had long ago considered that she would live for a long time. Yet the *potential* or *typical* physical toll of HIV still provided the language through which she expressed her experiences. "I'm not, like, 'Oh, I'm HIV,' you know? I believe God will take care of me. I don't have little routines or anything. I just, for the most part, try to forget that I'm HIV. It's not too hard to do that when you don't get side effects. I don't get any of that stuff like diarrhea. It's way on the back burner for me. Those medicines make that possible."

Similarly Jayla explained that her HIV is not the problem with which she most often deals; instead, she must face physical discomfort engendered by back surgery and cancer treatment. "I was told last my T cells is—my viral load is undetectable and my T cells is up around a thousand. Anyway, it's been undetectable for a long time. My HIV is not the problem. I got more things wrong with me than anyone should be allowed, and one of them is not my HIV. I got a hernia and chemo and diabetes and a bad back. They all worse than the HIV."

Jayla and Treva both felt that they were in good health as it related to HIV infection. Despite their favorable laboratory reports, both women continued to explain HIV disease in terms of physical symptoms. For Treva lacking symptoms that she considered typical for an HIV-positive person was a comfort. For Jayla her lack of HIV symptoms was a lens through which she could interpret the severity of other ailments she faced.

In addition to T cells and viral loads, precariously situated women's understandings of HIV disease focused on other tangible bodily signals, such as medication side effects, disease symptoms, and fatigue. Lisa, for example, explained living with HIV disease in terms of the physical effects of infection and of the laboratory analysis of the virus: "I'm undetectable and my T cells are up. That's been for a while now. He don't even take the blood but a few times a year, because I don't go in there with complaints. The only thing is that I'm having trouble sleeping. So when I go next, I'm gonna tell him about it. He'll help me out with that. Of course, though, I may have cervical cancer, so I have to go see my gynecologist this week too. I had abnormal cells in my Pap smear. They say HIV can do that. Now that's wild."

Lisa explained her experiences of HIV disease in terms of medical treatment and the course of the disease. Blood work, illness symptoms, and fatigue were just a few of the bodily processes that shaped her experiences of the disease. Similarly Tanya explained her experience in terms of the daily experience of immunodeficiency:

Just the daily struggle is hard. And it's getting to be wintertime, which is going to make it a lot harder. It's scarier during the wintertime because these little tiny sniffles can end up being a big deal. I was scared to death last year. I thought I was going to die. All that stuff was in the air. I had a bad cold. I lost my voice. I was stopped up. I was coughing really bad. I was, like, horrible. And you know, I just got really terrible, and it was hard because I know one day something like this will be the end of me. It's hard to know that something like a cold is going to kill you. People with HIV and AIDS die from everything.

As Tanya aptly stated, "it's hard to know" that common ailments may overburden a body taxed by immune dysfunction. This realization sometimes led to a kind of intense mindfulness concerning bodily distress signals. Colds were to be monitored. Chills and fevers had to be carefully treated. And in some cases the women's careful attention to their bodies averted impending AIDS-related illness. As Muriel described, "I know when it's [the virus] mutating—fever chills. That's when you know it's mutating. And I try to tell my doctor, 'Don't take away the bactrim.' That's when I need antibiotics, is when it's mutating. It pops my ears, I get muscle pains, and I'm irritable. It's a lot of stuff. You just take it one day at a time. It's all you can do. You learn to hear your body. You know when you going to get sick."

Muriel and Tanya's explanations of their HIV disease experience were similar to those of other precariously situated women in that the physicality of infection with the virus was emphasized over the emotional journey that stable women associated with infection. The declaration "you just take it one day at a time" was a common idiom that precariously situated women used to describe how unstable daily life conditions could be exacerbated or alleviated in relation to the physical aspects of infection. It was especially true for Peaches Q., a woman who had recently lost her son in a tragic shooting and was overburdened by a roach-infested apartment she could barely afford. Despite her intense grief and economic hardship, she felt optimistic because HIV disease was not yet threatening her physical health. "I mean, I have to be positive, you know. My, uh, CD4 level is way up. Blood pressure is under control. I'm taking my medicine for TB [tuberculosis] so it's what they call 'inactive' now. And, uh, I don't have to take medicine for HIV yet. So I don't have really any worries. I mean, I have stress, but as long as I don't get AIDS, I'm doing good."

While Peaches Q. was able to find a source of comfort in her HIV laboratory results during hardship, other women lamented their laboratory results in light of distress. Dana, for example, was distressed over her lack of social opportunities. Her family lived out of town, and only one sibling stayed in touch with her over the telephone. She was recently frightened to hear that her oldest brother had learned of her diagnosis as HIV-positive and had threatened to "come beat [her] ass for getting that shit."

Amid her fear of being beaten by her brother, Dana struggled to make ends meet. The chronic stress she faced intensified the auditory hallucinations she periodically experienced and her feeling that her life was most accurately characterized by worsening conditions. "I have real low T cells, and the other number is way too high. Can't something start going right for me? Nobody to talk to. My family won't even talk to me. No way to get anywhere. No money. And now I'm getting sick? I just feel like sometimes it couldn't get worse. And then it does."

Dana struggled to cope mentally with the circumstances of her life. Social isolation and economic hardship were daunting in and of themselves. Unfavorable HIV laboratory results became a prism of sorts through which she viewed the other hardships in her life. The immediacy of her multiple needs were brought into focus through her blood work.

Overall precariously situated women perceived HIV disease as a physical experience. Laboratory numbers indexing cellular changes, disease symptoms, and medication side effects provided the perceptual prism through which women in this group made sense of and discussed their survival with HIV disease. In the end their use of medical language can be interpreted as progress toward medical compliance and personal responsibility; however, they continued to be mired in present circumstances and preoccupations with the uncertainty of life rather than poised to strive toward future goals. In the specific context of HIV survival discourse, precariously situated women remained emotionally, educationally, and materially ill prepared to exhibit the "miracle" of the future promise on which the Treatment Modernization Act was built. Their realization of therapeutic citizenship therefore remained situational and contingent at best.

Vulnerable Women, Blood Work, and Perceptions of HIV Disease

Of all the women in this study, vulnerable women had the least obviously medical perceptions of HIV disease owing, at least in part, to the reality that they attended few events and meetings in the HIV-positive community. Their lack of attendance at community-sponsored events meant that vulnerable women had fewer opportunities for learning about and discussing an emotionally based or medically oriented perspective on life with the virus. Not attending such events was closely related to their strategies for survival.

Because vulnerable women relied heavily on personal social networks, disclosing their HIV status was a task fraught with fear of material deprivation. Disclosure was an especially salient issue for vulnerable women because they had few resources other than personal ties of mutual obligation; thus, revealing their HIV status potentially represented a severed tie with social network members. Calculating the potential risks and benefits of divulging one's HIV status was a serious business that had multiple dimensions with respect to the types of resources women foresaw losing should a disclosure process end unfavorably.

Many vulnerable women recalled disheartening disclosure experiences that left them without crucial resources. Consider, for example, Rachel's experience with disclosure to family members. Rachel was the legal guardian of her four children, two nieces, and one grandniece. When her mother died, she moved from North Carolina to be near an aunt in Indiana who had offered to help raise the children. A week after her arrival, Rachel told her aunt that she was HIV-positive. Her aunt's reaction was unfavorable. Rachel explained, "When I confided in her, she went the other way with it. She said that I wasn't fit to raise those kids. I needed to give up my rights to them and give the rights to her because there was no telling how long I would be around. The youngest one was six at the time, and she was telling me that there was no way I was going to see him grown and 'you know this, so face the facts.' She just turned on me and made an appointment with a lawyer."

Rachel described how her aunt had assumed that she was unfit to raise the children because of her HIV-positive status. Fearful of losing custody of the children, Rachel fled her aunt's house with the children in the middle of the night. She left behind all of her belongings, including clothing, furniture, and personal items. She and the children made it back to North Carolina with the help of an Indiana Salvation Army program. She soon relinquished the children to Social Services, however, because she was unable to provide them a fit home environment. Although it all happened more than twelve years prior to our interviews, Rachel had not yet recovered the relative material stability she had once had. At the time of our second interview, she had been actually homeless for more than a year and technically homeless for two years. She was still unable to afford replacement furniture, clothing, and other such items that make an apartment or home habitable. This experience with disclosure left Rachel wary of broaching the subject with other loved ones and friends.

In addition to material hardship, the disclosure of one's HIV-positive status carried the potential threat of physical violence. This possibility was true for study participants in all socioeconomic groups, as Dana's experience with her brother attests. For vulnerable women, however, the violence related to disclosure was more commonly realized and egregious. Tasha recalled a murder related to a disclosure experience she had witnessed on "the avenue," where sex work transactions were frequent. She said, "I seen this girl get stoned to death. This guy hit her in the head with a cement block because she was out there selling her body and she had told him that she was HIV so they had to use condoms. But, see, I don't see why this guy got so mad because he was the one who didn't want to use any condoms and she was honest. . . . He threw a cement block and crushed her skull. She died right there."

Witnessing the murder of her acquaintance was, of course, traumatic. As a result she was "extremely careful" when deciding with whom she might discuss her condition. Likewise, Chantelle was cautious about disclosing to men in particular. She sometimes feared that her HIV-positive status would bring her to a fate similar to what Tasha had witnessed. A man Chantelle had previously "run with" learned of her infection and began threatening her. He told her to "sleep with one eye open" at the shelters because he planned to "rape her dirty ass." Chantelle said, "He say, 'I'm a sneak in your room tonight, and you can't lock your door.' It don't bother me because I got a kitchen knife out of my friend's kitchen. I sleep with it under my pillow. I say, 'I'm waiting on you because I can cut the rest of that little bitty nasty thing off. You be running around, and we call you Nubby then.'" Despite Chantelle's mocking assertion that she could defend herself, she remained careful about revealing her status to others.

In addition to violence, disclosure sometimes resulted in vulnerable women being extorted by their peers. As Georgia explained, "Well, like, one girl I told, and then she told this other girl even though I told her not to. And then that girl—she would start asking me for stuff like cigarettes and whatever, and when I didn't want to give her none, she called me a 'AIDS-carrying bitch.' Sometimes if there was people around, I had to give her my stuff or else then everybody would know. So I stopped telling anybody. Don't tell just anybody and especially not nobody who will use it over you."

Georgia's experiences with being intimidated were tinged with regret for ever having disclosed her status to individuals she could not, in the end, trust. Being called an AIDS-carrying bitch was not only an attack on her sense of self-worth but also a means of further revealing Georgia's HIV status to others within earshot of the altercation. This type of disclosure threatened to ostracize Georgia from her personal social network, further complicating her strategies for achieving daily life stability and satisfying basic needs.

Chantelle also had an experience where unintentional disclosure left her disconnected from her social network. Chantelle, however, bought her way back into her social circle by providing drugs and alcohol to her friends. As she described,

> At first I wanted to kill myself because everybody knew. And when it get around that "she has AIDS" and when they seen me coming, they shut up. I said, "Well, the only way you going to be my friend is if I buy liquor and crack, and I'll do that." Because I was very lonely even though I'm not alone in this disease, but at the time I felt very lonely, depressed—like I just lost my best friend. You know? It was killing me, and I thought, "Why shouldn't I just go ahead and kill myself now?" And I was suicidal because I was so depressed and alone.

Although Chantelle was able to maintain her social ties to friends by furnishing them with crack and alcohol, she continued to feel isolated and distant from her peers. Her depression worsened, and she soon began devising ways to end her life. In the course of two years, she attempted suicide more than five times. She swallowed large amounts of pills. She jumped in front of cars on the highway. And she tried nightly to drink herself to death until 2009 when she achieved temporary sobriety for three months. Chantelle's experiences with disclosure, on all accounts, had failed to produce favorable results.

When asked to discuss the effects of HIV on their lives, vulnerable women explained the potential and actual effects that infection and disclosure had on their social networks and relationships. Tasha, for example, described living with the virus as hell because

> I just think you a outcast. Yeah, I still feel that way. Outcast and especially if somebody finds out. Even my closest friends and the girl that's a female that I felt really close with, I didn't tell her because one day

she made a comment like, "I heard she got that shit." She was talking about somebody else. Why would I tell her? You going to think the same thing about me, so she don't even know. Yeah, you do feel alone. They say, "Go to, like, support groups," and stuff like that, but trust me, you still feel alone. All they do is tell everybody your business.

Tasha explained that HIV disease set her apart from her peers. Women whose lives and livelihoods depended on their peers acutely felt the social stigma associated with the virus. While all of the women in this study acknowledged that the stigma of HIV disease partially shaped their disclosure decisions, vulnerable women were the only participants who discussed this stigma as materially and socially devastating.

Rosalind and Amanda further explained that HIV disease was most burdensome in terms of its effects on their social lives. For Rosalind, the stigmatization of HIV disease posed difficulties in everyday social interactions. She explained her experience this way: "It's hard because you feel like people look at you and know that you got it. And that's where you need strength to act like you ain't got it so that you're not acting funny when people talk about it or are looking at you like you got it." Amanda also explained HIV disease as socially difficult. She, however, emphasized social abandonment: "To me, this disease is like drama and stress. Not being able to tell everybody. Having to keep it a secret. You have to because some people still haven't got the idea that they're not going to catch it just from being around you. They think it's so deadly that they leave you the second they find out."

For vulnerable women such as Tasha, Rosalind, and Amanda, HIV disease perhaps most importantly represented an affront to their social relationships. Ostracism was an emotional and material toll they feared and sometimes paid as a consequence of infection with a stigmatized virus. For them laboratory testing and physical symptoms were of less immediate consequence than their potentially and actually disrupted social networks were.

When I probed vulnerable women to discuss their laboratory blood work and physical experience with the disease, their responses highlighted a lack of certainty regarding the particulars of HIV infection and medical surveillance. Some vulnerable women declared they did not want to learn the language of HIV care as taught through service programs. "I know all I want to. . . . Take medicine. That's all you need," Donna explained. Other women, like Rachel, felt that HIV-related education was overwhelming given its evolving nature. She asserted, "There's always more [to learn]. You never done because they're [doctors] always learning. . . . I want to know more, but where do you start?" In any case, the women's lack of medical knowledge concerning HIV blood work and viral infection was reinforced by their precarious attachment to the system of HIV care and their lack of participation in affiliated pedagogical exercises.

Given this situation, vulnerable women seemed to little understand the common terminology that care providers used when assessing their health. The women linked the phrases "CD4 cell count" and "viral load" with laboratory testing numbers, but they were unsure as to the relevance of those numbers for health. When asked about their most current laboratory analyses, vulnerable women sometimes responded with explanations of factors they felt were more important than laboratory work. For example, Chantelle said,

> With my doctor, he tells me a summary of the lab works. I piece [it] together—it's not what he's saying that I listen to. It's what he's not saying. . . . I read between the lines. . . . So when he talks about medication or HIV, I hear that I am healthy because then he send me down to the lab and we draw some blood and that's no problem. He does a small physical and it don't last long and I'm out the door. If it were longer, I might be worried and reading something else out of it.

Instead of interpreting the numerical language of laboratory diagnostics, Chantelle relied on the routine nature of physician visits to tell her what she needed to know about her health. Other vulnerable women prioritized their doctors' qualitative assessments of their health, sometimes assuming unlikely relationships between perceived symptoms and what laboratory numbers may indicate. Rosalind explained that "I worry all the time that my head is shrinking and it means I'm going to die. Then my doctor looks at my paper and tells me that my labs look good, so I guess my head shrinking means the medicine is working."

While some vulnerable women explained this kind of indirect use of laboratory analyses, others more specifically admitted that they did not really understand what the laboratory numbers meant. In a conversation about her health, Rachel stated, "I don't know [about my health] as far as the number wise. I have a appointment next week, and I said that I was going start asking my doctor to help me with it because everybody always asking me."

Donna similarly explained, "I don't know about those numbers. I just go by how I feel. I was feeling fine so I stopped my medication, but the doctor said it don't work like that. I got to keep taking it. I was on two pills, but now I'm on four because I guess I messed it all up." Thus Donna's not understanding the HIV laboratory work led her to rely solely on detecting disease symptoms for her self-health assessment. Her experience illustrates how in vulnerable women's estimations, CD4 cell count and viral load numbers fell under the purview of physicians and employees of programmatic services. Vulnerable women had little material advantage in understanding and using the language of laboratory results, particularly given their persistent ineligibility for support service programs. Learning the language of blood work, however, could have possibly provided a social bridge between the vulnerable women and those care providers who were skeptical of their efforts to comply with institutional norms and guidelines.

Blood Work and Biosocial Inclusion

Women's experiences with the blood-work mandate shed light on federally funded HIV/AIDS care as a therapeutic site shaped by values commensurate with a market-based model of governance. Here the personal responsibility for one's living conditions and health circumstances saddled the women with specific burdens of self-care, including the imperative to understand and address HIV/AIDS in biomedical terms. Midway's system of care in this way offered therapeutic intervention on two counts: federally funded HIV/AIDS care services allocated medically oriented programs for individuals living with HIV disease; and at the same time it taught socially marginal women to assume a biologically mediated social identity characterized by their HIV-positive status and their willingness to submit themselves to biomedical disease management practices. By itself the blood-work mandate represents another means for understanding the "neoliberalization of HIV health care" insofar as it required socially marginal women to subscribe to logics of disease underpinned by notions of cost efficiency, of individualism, and of assuming the personal responsibility to realize a life productively lived.

Meanwhile clearly the women in this study conceptualized and expressed their feelings concerning the bodily experience of HIV infection differently. While all of the women had some access to the language of biomedicine via state-required blood work, the relevance of that language was shaped by the women's daily life circumstances. In other words, the blood-work mandate did not operate in socially uniform ways across this population of women. Instead, it articulated with existing material and social inequalities in ways that amplified the varied structural positions shaping their engagement with state-sanctioned perspectives on blood work, health, and survival with HIV disease. Differential use of the biomedical language of CD4 cell and viral load testing thus signified the contingent nature of biosocial inclusion in this context.

This analysis of the women's varied degrees of consonance with the language and perspective of laboratory diagnostics reveals some contradictions and inconsistencies of biosocial inclusion in this HIV/AIDS care context. Laboratory testing was obligatory for all of the women, yet only precariously situated women viewed it as a reliable and singularly important source of health information. While their compliance with medical directives to complete regular laboratory work was conducive to program eligibility, their reliance on the numbers reported in laboratory diagnostics was paradoxically inappropriate in relation to the broader dictates of a survival discourse focused on the future. Instead of narrowing their concerns to immediate and present conditions of health, care providers sought to instill in these women a sense of the long-term future. Women who clung tightly to the numbers, who did not understand the numbers, or who could not produce "good" numbers clearly had not yet internalized that the "miracle" of "free" HIV/AIDS care somehow implied their personal responsibility of not needing it in the future.

Stable women, in contrast, understood blood work was situational and, most important, only partially constitutive of the realities of their HIV health. Testing sensitivity, timing, and personal health circumstances factored into the numbers they received from physicians. They understood that small drops in CD4 cell counts and incremental rises in viral loads were perhaps problems of science and technology. Service providers could interpret this view as a positive step toward not "using lab work as a lifestyle," as Natasha put it, meaning that stable women indeed seized their capacity to represent "the future promise" of this "public health miracle." HIV would thus not represent a barrier to motivation, future plans, and self-sufficiency. In an important way stable women freed themselves from the emotional stress that anxiety concerning laboratory analysis sometimes involved. They also freed themselves from the self-doubt that can sometimes accompany chronic health concerns. In another way, however, stable women firmly entrenched themselves in individualizing processes of biomedicine that left them without a language of redress when the resources they used failed to put right the inequalities and barriers that shaped their infection in the first place.

Conclusion

LIFE BEYOND SURVIVAL

When I returned to the field in 2012, I learned many women in this study had disassociated themselves from Health Partnership. In a few cases the severing of this institutional connection was a positive development. Charlotte, for example, was the home owner she had long planned to be. She was also well on her way to having a state license to practice as a drug addiction counselor. In the meantime she continued to receive monthly disability checks in addition to a small stipend for her part-time work as a counseling intern at a local grassroots antipoverty agency. Tamara, I heard, had worked through many of the emotional issues she faced concerning her HIV-positive diagnosis and, having long been financially stable, felt she no longer needed the kind of support Health Partnership had to offer. Stacey, although still in need of public support services, had enrolled in a program for substance abusers who had achieved long-term sobriety. She no longer lived in the recovery house because she had secured her own apartment. I last visited her in that apartment, a place she felt represented the beginning of a new life chapter for her. I was surprised to learn in 2013 that she died in the hospital, having been very sick for a protracted time.

Other women still needed regular access to support services but chose not to utilize Health Partnership because agency protocol had grown increasingly restrictive and, in their experiences, had become demeaning. Joan and Lisa, for example, both described Health Partnership in 2012 as "having changed," and they referred to new rules that disallowed hanging out at the agency or stopping by in hopes of securing a walk-in appointment. For Joan the decision to disconnect ultimately meant that she received the bulk of her support services from an agency serving the needs of Midway's poor, regardless of their HIV status. This agency contracted with Medicaid, so it technically also received federal funding for HIV/AIDS services provision. In her estimation close relationships and volunteer work with care providers at this other agency continued to bolster her chances for support.

Lisa, in contrast, found herself increasingly far afield from the community built around the local HIV/AIDS epidemic or any community, for that matter. Long days spent alone were punctuated by long nights spent sharing alcohol and drugs with neighbors she otherwise barely knew. She felt her decision to drop Health Partnership was ultimately self-preserving, but she lamented being "being alone" and "far from anyone who knew about her conditions." Not being connected to other agencies and other women living with similar health circumstances ultimately diminished her resource base and social network opportunities. Social isolation was a challenge Lisa had long sought to avoid. She was intensely friendly and endeavored to connect with others wherever she went; thus her disconnection from Health Partnership was difficult for her on many fronts. When her daughters informed me that she had died in the summer of 2014, I hoped she had not been alone.

Still other women, such as Muriel, Treva, and Tanya, were officially "lost to care"; that is, care providers were unsure whether they were enrolled in services anywhere or were even still alive. A local hospital hired Natasha to find clients who were lost to care in an effort to reestablish contact and services. Natasha's sense was that despite her best efforts, the women would remain out of contact until they chose to reconnect. No one was sure at that time whether upcoming changes to federal health care policy would have any impact on the women's willingness to reengage with care or on the availability of Midway's public HIV/AIDS programs. Care providers seemed to anticipate another slate of potentially disorienting public health policy changes.

Health Partnership remained in operation, of course. It continued to funnel Ryan White CARE Act dollars into the community, and its employees still battled the epidemic one client at a time. While some employees with whom I managed to reconnect wondered aloud what lost-to-care and successful clients were up to, the reality was that new clients had come to take their place. Few employees had time to ponder the where-abouts, the progress, or the disappointments of clients who no longer used or needed their services. Moreover, agency newcomers had replaced many Health Partnership employees who are featured in this study. As Myra, one of the few remaining employees who had participated in my research, put it, "They cleaned house. Even [the executive director] left. It's just gotten really hard and really scary around here. Like, I'm wor-ried about if I'm going to have a job if this health care reform goes through." Indeed, the landscape of local Ryan White–funded care will continue to change in response to shifting American political and eco-nomic circumstances.

Lived Experiences of Health Policy

Holding On thus represents a moment captured along a longer timeline of political economic processes; it is an ethnography of public health policy as southern, HIV-positive African American women enrolled in federally funded HIV/AIDS care experienced it in the post–Treatment Modernization Act era. At the outset of this research in 2007, African American women constituted 72 percent of *all* reported HIV/AIDS cases in the South (Fullilove 2006, 11). Although federally funded HIV/AIDS-care programs had long sought to enhance their access to and retention in care by targeting health care and socioeconomic support services to them USDHHS 2014), they remained at greater risk for poor HIV-related health (CDC 2015). The experiences recounted here shed light on this persistent unequal distribution of risk for poor HIV-related health by tracing complexities of access to public health care resources.

Principal among complexities of access to health resources was the transformation of Ryan White CARE Act programs. Ryan White CARE was no longer about "keeping the lights on" or addressing the daily life needs of clients, as an agency employee once explained. It was instead about igniting behavioral change among a population popularly believed to be socially and morally deficient. In effect, then, policy changes to Ryan White legislation realigned federally funded HIV/AIDS care accord-ing to values associated with economic development. Decreasing funds for HIV-specific antipoverty programs and increasing requirements con-cerning medical surveillance and behavior change ensured that federally funded HIV/AIDS care could scarcely be seen as a fiscally "inefficient," "anti–free market," or "immoral" public health intervention.

At the local level legislative changes moved health-related agencies and service providers, such as those at Health Partnership, to demonstrate their compliance with moral logics of cost-effectiveness and personal responsibility. However unintentionally in this way the 2006 TMA and the 2009 Treatment Extension Act stimulated new forms and contexts for disseminating and performing values of neoliberalism and, in the process, generated new forms of social marginalization and empowerment (Biehl 2007; Comaroff and Comaroff 2001; Susser 2009). The HIV-positive women navigated these changing terrains of HIV/AIDS care and claimed nonmedical support in a context otherwise characterized by the retrenchment of social welfare services.

However, the women's experiences of service use were varied and complex. They belied the idea that HIV-positive status confers on programmatic service users the kind of biosocial inclusion documented in other parts of the world. In some cases the women's support claims relied directly on exploiting the social differences among themselves, a move that, as highlighted here, spotlights policy as a critical pathway by which health inequalities proliferate. Resulting distinctions in the women's eligibility for HIV/AIDS-related services in Midway were demarcated around moral categories driven by health care policies concerned with medical and social surveillance, with controlling feelings of entitlement to state support, and, in the context of community volunteer work, with facilitating productivity (see also Bourgois 2000). Thus care providers and those women who were well positioned in the care continuum considered some support claims as legitimate while others could only be seen as pathological. Here the concept of personal responsibility underpinned novel means of difference making vis-à-vis a moral economy based on an ethnographically specific notion of survival.

Survival

In the context of the federally funded system of HIV/AIDS care, survival represented far more than an epidemiological measure concerning a person's length of life and disease prognosis. Indeed, in related contexts of medical advancement, global capitalism, and the divestment of antipoverty programs, the notion of survival was infused with an informal responsibility to earn the "privilege" of "free" HIV/AIDS health care and supportive services by recovering or correcting one's life. Ryan White CARE Act amendments and reauthorization bills drew on metaphors such as "getting it together" and the "miracle" of Ryan White CARE to convey an important shift in the realities of services provision. Gone were the days of certain death and thus a system charged solely with administrating palliative care. Contemporary realities of medical advancement and a growing popular disdain for welfare dependency spurred a new generation of HIV/AIDS care programming aimed at safeguarding the productivity of otherwise healthy HIV-positive citizens and the rehabilitation of individuals who lost their footing on the path to self-sufficiency. This shift occurred at the same time that Ryan White CARE Act programming began restricting funding for and access to ancillary services. In other words, the women in this study were charged with the difficult task of demonstrating daily life stability and their prioritization of HIV health at the same time that their resource base for doing so diminished.

Even though many care providers recognized the material uncertainties shaping their clients' lives, they often faced ambiguities in policy language and agency protocol. In these instances, they tended to interpret their jobs and service mandates in relation to broader trends associated with welfare reform. The predominant discourses of dependence and deservingness shaped care providers' understanding that they were disciplining a population "used to getting something for nothing," as Greg put it. They thus required the women to convey their consonance with the values undergirding new conditions of survival as a criterion of receiving services. In Midway's system of care, these values included locally inflected notions of personal responsibility as well as the adoption of a biomedically savvy perspective on HIV disease and related diagnostics. Survival thus shaped and prioritized particular kinds of knowledge and experience concerning what it means to live with HIV disease. It also provided the basis for a service provision hierarchy among a socially diverse group of African American women.

For some women, survival was profoundly disempowering as they did not fulfill the implied imperative to adopt the predominant understanding of HIV disease as a chronic health condition with which they could move forward in life. They continued to live, but their lives could not be used as a testament to the "legacy of care" built by the Ryan White CARE Act. Survival for them involved, in part, the daily experience of being excluded from services and of struggling to fulfill material needs and wants.

For other women, however, their survival was at least sometimes productive as a cultural resource through which they could gain increased access to services and Health Partnership personnel. Their lives dramatized survival in an elaborated sense of restoring or gaining a life well lived and thus highlighted the efficacy of federally funded health care services. Paradoxically their ability to convey self-regulation granted increased access to the regulatory and therapeutic services of Health Partnership. In this way, survival was neither simply a continued state of being in the world nor solely an expression of agency amid formidable constraint nor, ironically, the utilization of unsanctioned means for satisfying basic needs. Survival was instead a mechanism of social inclusion and material deservingness. In an ethnographically specific way, survival with HIV disease operated for the women in this study as a means for turning the constraints of health care reform into possibilities for moral belonging and realities of material advancement.

Public Health Futures

This ethnographic account of survival among poor Black women living with HIV/AIDS has much to teach about success and failure in public health policy and programs. To the credit of legislators, care providers, and the women themselves, all study participants were enrolled and participated in health care. Every woman in this study had at least technical access to life-saving medications and medical care. Additionally many women in this study recovered and/or maintained their health using the services, tools, and advice provided through the administration of Ryan White CARE Act funds. In this way the legacy of Ryan White–funded care is indeed profoundly life affirming.

However, the women's experiences with disease management in contexts of poverty and federally funded HIV/AIDS care dramatize the shortcomings of contemporary health policy in informative ways. Perhaps first and foremost, while public health officials, legislators, and activists have long focused on increasing access to medical treatment for HIV/ AIDS, attention to contexts of health and survival has dwindled. Antiretroviral therapy may be widely available, medical appointment copayments may be covered, and counselors may be well trained to provide therapeutic services; however, the lesson remains: access to health care is a multidimensional issue that is intractably tethered to material conditions of daily life. *Holding On* refocuses our attention on the interplay between living conditions and health needs by examining how subtle differences among the women translated into not-so-subtle differences in support service access. It also refocuses our attention on relationships between social inequality and HIV health disparity. This fine-grained analysis of variability among a population of HIV-positive Black women highlights how social performance, moral consonance, and material advantage structure access to health resources.

Finally this study dramatizes the dynamism between health policy and daily life experience. We see through an ethnographic lens how policy has shaped the realities of the women's lives. We also see, however, how both the women and the care providers enacted and acted on health policy in ways that ultimately defined what the Treatment Modernization Act may be said to do.

This dynamic perspective on survival with HIV/AIDS encourages anthropologists, public health officials, and public health practitioners to consider the political, economic, social, and emotional dimensions of life with chronic infectious disease. In the particular case of the women in Midway, a one-size-fits-all approach to health services delivery was problematic. Varied circumstances of housing, finances, legal status, mental health, and chemical dependency differentially affected the women's abilities to utilize programs theoretically designed for "hard-to-reach" populations. The fine details of life, in other words, mattered in important ways for using health services. As we move forward in our response to the continuing story of HIV/AIDS care and the tenuous circumstances of women who are holding on for dear life, policies and programmatic services must pay heed to the diverse conditions of social circumstance and daily life.

Appendix 1

Demographic Characteristics of Study Participants at Time of First Interview

Table 1. Study participants' demographic information

	MONTHLY INCOME	MAJOR INCOME SOURCES	HOUSING STATUS/PAYMENT	SUBSTANCE USE STATUS	MARITAL STATUS	EDUCATION	YEAR OF HIV DIAGNOSIS	AGE
Amanda	$0	None	Recovery house/$0	In recovery	Separated	GED	2007	42
Andrea	$0	None	Renter/family pays	Declined to discuss	Never married	9th grade	2000	45
Ashley	$1,400	SSI, employment	Renter/$300	Never used drugs	Never married	11th grade	2000	Late 50s
Brenda	$1,452	SSI, survivor's benefits	Renter/$580	Never used drugs	Never married	11th grade	2006	34
Chantelle	$0	No source of cash income	Homeless	Active addiction	Widowed	GED	2000	45
Charlotte	$950	SSI, SSDI	Renter/$140	Long-term recovery	Divorced	Some college	1999	51
Christina	$860–$875	SSDI, odd jobs	Renter/$475	In recovery	Never married	11th grade	2001	33
Dana	$637	SSDI	Renter/$320	In recovery	Never married	7th grade	Early 1990s	49
Danielle	$657	SSDI	Renter/$161	Never used drugs	Divorced	11th grade	Early 1990s	68
Debdai	$600	SSDI, survivor's benefits	Renter/$82	Never used drugs	Never married	High school diploma	2000	45

	MONTHLY INCOME	MAJOR INCOME SOURCES	HOUSING STATUS/PAYMENT	SUBSTANCE USE STATUS	MARITAL STATUS	EDUCATION	YEAR OF HIV DIAGNOSIS	AGE
DeeDee	$1,167–$1,867	Military pension, temporary work	Cares for mother in family home/ approx. $200	In recovery	Never married	Some college	1999	48
Donna	$416	Part-time CNA work	Technically homeless	Declined to discuss	Never married	10th grade	1999	49
Elizabeth	$1,000	Odd jobs, spouse	Renter/$425	Active addiction	Married	High school diploma	1997	42
Georgia	$30–$40	Odd jobs	Technically homeless	Active addiction	Never married	11th grade	1998	44
Grace	Approximately $1,400	SSDI, pension	Renter/$630	Never used drugs	Divorced	Bachelor's degree	2004	51
Jamie	$0	None	Technically homeless	Trying for recovery	Divorced, widowed	High school diploma	2000	43
Jayla	$637	SSDI	Renter/$250	Never used drugs	Separated	High school diploma	1991	50
Joan	$950	SSDI, SSI	Renter/$120	Never used drugs	Married	Some college	1993	33
Kareese	$745	SSDI	Renter/$325 split with husband	In recovery	Married	10th grade	2000	37
Karen	$643	SSDI, SSI	Renter/$52	In recovery	Never married	High school diploma	1985	48

	Income	Income source	Housing	Substance use	Marital status	Education	Year	Age
Lady E.	$250 until SSDI approved ($650)	Small business, welfare until SSDI approved	Renter/$435 per month	In recovery	Never married	College degree	1993	49
Lessa	$636	SSDI	Renter/$325	Active addiction	Separated	10th grade	2000	52
Linda	$900–$1,725	Employment, survivor's benefits	Renter/$850	Never used drugs	Widowed	Some college	1998	40s
Lisa	$723	SSDI, stipend for non-profit work	Renter/$475	Intermittent recovery, active addiction	Never married	Some college	1993	50
Marjorie	$200–$900	Temporary work	Renter/$150	Never used drugs	Never married	High school diploma	2002	32
Muriel	$546	Disability	Renter/$127	Active addiction	Never married	11th grade	1987	45
Noelle	$726	SSI, VA pension	Renter/$350	In recovery	Widowed	11th grade	1994	42
Peaches Q.	$900	SSDI of husband, employment	Renter/$300	Never used drugs	Married	12th grade (no diploma)	2005	50
Rachel	$563	SSDI	Homeless	In recovery	Never married	10th grade	1995	Early 50s
Raquel	$645	SSDI	Renter/$375	Active addiction	Never married	7th grade	Unsure, prior to 1998	47

	MONTHLY INCOME	MAJOR INCOME SOURCES	HOUSING STATUS/PAYMENT	SUBSTANCE USE STATUS	MARITAL STATUS	EDUCATION	YEAR OF HIV DIAGNOSIS	AGE
Rene	$600	SSDI	Renter/$127	Long-term recovery	Never married	4th grade	1990	59
Rosalind	$0	None	Technically homeless	Never used drugs	Never married	High school diploma	2006	53
Samantha	$694	SSDI	Renter/$550	Active addiction	Married	10th grade	1993	43
Sharon	$500	SSDI	Technically homeless/$250	Active addiction	Divorced	10th grade	1999	45
Shayna	$656	SSDI	Renter/$375	In recovery	Never married	11th grade	Early 1990s	51
Stacey	$637	SSI	Renter/$0 through program	In recovery	Never married	Associate degree	1991	50
Tamara	Declined to be specific; finances indicated as "middle class"	Husband's income	Home owner/payment not specified	Never used drugs	Married	High school diploma	2004	42
Tanya	$100 until employed ($930)	Employment	Renter/$0 until employed ($425)	Never used drugs	Married	High school diploma	Early 2000s	26
Tasha	$900	Disability	Homeless	Active addiction	Never married	Diploma	1996	47
Treva	$623	SSDI	Renter/$450	In recovery	Married	11th grade	1990	47

Appendix 2

Study Participants' Analytic Categories

Table 2. Stable women

	MONTHLY INCOME	RENT AS % OF INCOME	"DISPOSABLE" INCOME (AFTER AVERAGE BASIC HOME BILLS $241)
Ashley	$1,400	21	$859
Charlotte	$950	15	$569
Danielle	$657	25	$255
Debdai	$600	14	$277
DeeDee	$1,167, plus varied temp income	17	$726, plus temp income
Grace	$1,400 (payee)	45	$529
Joan	$950	13	$589
Stacey	$637	0	$396
Tamara	Not specified	Not specified	Not available

Table 3. Precariously situated women

	MONTHLY INCOME	RENT AS % OF INCOME	"DISPOSABLE" INCOME (AFTER AVERAGE BASIC HOME BILLS $241)
Brenda	$1,452	40	$631
Christina	$875	54	$159
Dana	$637	50	$317, utilities included in rent
Jayla	$637	39	$146
Kareese	$745	44	$179
Karen	$643	8	$350
Lady E.	$650	67	–$26
Lessa	$636 (payee)	51	$70
Linda	$1,725	49	$634
Lisa	$723	66	$7
Marjorie	$200–$900 (variable)	75–17	Varied, depending on income; utilities included in rent
Muriel	$546	23	$178
Noelle	$726	48	$135
Peaches Q.	$900	33	$359
Raquel	$645 (payee)	58	$29
Rene	$600	21	$232
Samantha	$694	79	-$97
Shayna	$656	57	$40
Tanya	$930	46	$264
Treva	$623	72	–$68

Table 4. Vulnerable women

	MONTHLY INCOME	RENT AS % OF INCOME	"DISPOSABLE" INCOME (AFTER AVERAGE BASIC HOME BILLS $241)
Amanda	$0	Recovery house	$0
Andrea	$0	Family pays rent temporarily	No cash
Chantelle	$0	Homeless	Any cash earned goes to potential host
Donna	$416 (until job lost)	Technically homeless, no rent	Any cash earned goes to utilities
Elizabeth	$1,000 (variable spousal income)	43	$334 (controlled by spouse)
Georgia	$40	Technically homeless	Cash goes to household
Jamie	$0	Technically homeless, though in a secure relationship	$0
Rachel	$563	Homeless	$563
Rosalind	$0	Technically homeless	$0
Sharon	$500	Technically homeless; 50% goes to brother	Extra cash goes to host for utilities and food
Tasha	$900	Homeless	Extra cash goes to potential host, hotel rooms

Appendix 3

Glossary of Service Program Acronyms

ADAP (AIDS Drug Assistance Program): In North Carolina the AIDS Drug
Assistance Program uses a combination of state and federal funds to
provide low-income residents with access to HIV/AIDS medications,
including medications designed to treat the opportunistic infections
associated with the virus (U.S. Department of Health and Human
Services [USDHHS] 2009c).

AFDC (Aid to Families with Dependent Children): AFDC was a federal income
assistance program for children and the families of unemployed parents.
The program was originally outlined in Title IV of the 1935 Social Security
Act. It existed until 1995, when the government dismantled it as a part of
the 1996 welfare reform efforts of the Clinton era (U.S. Census Bureau
2011).

CRCS (Comprehensive Risk Counseling and Services): CRCS is a federally
funded program designed to be an intensive, individual-level risk
reduction and intervention service. Program participants meet with a risk
reduction counselor for individual consultations and counseling sessions.
The primary goal of the service is to reduce the chances of HIV infection
and transmission among individuals who are considered to be at high
risk. The program was formerly known as "prevention case management"
(Centers for Disease Control 2009).

EBT (electronic benefits transfer): EBT refers to the state nutritional assistance
program, also known as food stamps. Participants receive a plastic card,
much like a credit card, that allows them to spend the "food stamp
money" deposited each month in their account (North Carolina Division
of Social Services 2009).

FEMA (Federal Emergency Management Agency): FEMA is a federal agency
charged with the task of mitigating disaster and coordinating recovery
programs associated with disaster. FEMA created the Emergency Food and
Shelter National Board Program in 1983 to supplement the work of local

social service organizations in the United States. This program provides food and money, allocated by states, for the support of homeless and food-insecure populations (Federal Emergency Management Agency 2015).

HOPWA (Housing Opportunities for People with AIDS): HOPWA is a federal program that provides grants to states and cities for a variety of services, including housing assistance for HIV-positive populations. The funds can be used for the acquisition, rehabilitation, or new construction of housing units; costs for housing facility operations; rental assistance for individuals living with HIV/AIDS; and short-term payments to prevent homelessness (U.S. Department of Housing and Urban Development 2009).

PRWORA (Personal Responsibility and Work Opportunity Reconciliation Act): PRWORA is a comprehensive welfare reform bill that Congress enacted in 1996. Essentially the bill dismantled AFDC and replaced it with the Temporary Assistance for Needy Families (TANF) program. The broader bill contains work requirements that mandate welfare recipients to work in exchange for their benefits after two years of enrollment and imposes a lifetime limit of benefits receipt equal to five years. The bill also provides performance bonuses to reward states for moving welfare recipients into paid jobs, and it stipulates additional child care funding for eligible families and health care coverage for recipients, including one year of Medicaid coverage when participants leave welfare for work.

In addition PWORA mandates comprehensive child support enforcement, including an executive action to track "delinquent parents" across state lines. The law expanded wage garnishment, allowed states to seize assets and require community service, and to revoke drivers' licenses from parents who owe delinquent child support (USDHHS 2009d).

Ryan White CARE Act (Ryan White Comprehensive AIDS Resources Emergency Act): First authorized in 1990, the Ryan White CARE Act provides the impetus for federal support of HIV/AIDS health care and related programs. The Ryan White program works with cities, states, and local community-based organizations to provide services for HIV-positive individuals who do not have sufficient health care coverage or financial resources for managing the disease (USDHHS 2009c).

SNAP (State Nutritional Assistance Program): Since 1997 SNAP has provided funds for North Carolina central food distribution centers. The central distribution centers use the funds to purchase staple foods in bulk from North Carolina companies. In turn, these staple foods are distributed to area food banks, rescue missions, soup kitchens, and various types of publicly funded shelters (Food Bank of Central and Eastern North Carolina 2009).

SSDI (Social Security Disability Insurance): SSDI is a federal program for people with disabilities who are unable to work. The program pays benefits to individuals who have a qualifying disability and who have paid a qualifying amount in Social Security taxes. Qualifying disabilities include medical conditions that result in the inability to perform work and/or that are expected to last at least one year or result in death. Individuals accumulate Social Security work credits based on total yearly wages, with a maximum of four credits earned each year (equivalent to earning $4,480). Individuals who have accumulated forty credits, twenty of which were earned in the ten years prior to the onset of the disability, qualify for the program (Social Security Administration 2009).

SSI (Supplemental Security Insurance): SSI is a federal income support program that is funded by general taxes (not Social Security). Disabled individuals who have limited income and resources can qualify for this program. Payments are based on financial need. SSDI payments are included as a resource in SSI eligibility calculations (Social Security Administration 2009).

TANF (Temporary Assistance for Needy Families): Under the welfare reform legislation (PWRORA) of 1996, TANF replaced the welfare programs known as AFDC, the Job Opportunities and Basic Skills training program, and the Emergency Financial Assistance (EFA) Program. The law ended federal entitlement to assistance and instead created TANF as a block grant that provides federal funds to states, territories, and tribes each year. These funds cover benefits, administrative expenses, and services targeted to poor families (USDHHS 2009a).

TEFAP (The Emergency Food Assistance Program): Under 1996 welfare reform, TEFAP and the Soup Kitchen/U.S. Department of Agriculture (USDA) Commodities have been merged into one program. Administered by the state, TEFAP funds are used to purchase food for low-income populations. The food is distributed through emergency assistance agencies and other charities for registered clients (Food Bank of Central and Eastern North Carolina 2009).

TMA (Treatment Modernization Act): The TMA amended and reauthorized the Ryan White CARE Act in 2006 and 2009. The guidelines, in general, serve to reprioritize funding levels for different states. Southern states have received significantly more federal dollars than they had in years past. North Carolina, in particular, received a $6.5 million increase in funding for the fiscal year 2007.

Funding level increases for southern states ushered in new regulations about how Ryan White money can be spent. In the South, adding new programs for substance abuse recovery, behavioral interventions, and medical care were a priority. In fact, 75 percent of all Ryan White funds were specifically targeted to core medical services, including physician appointments, prescription programs, and medical adherence counseling (USDHHS 2009b).

VR (vocational rehabilitation): VR is a state program that is administered through the North Carolina Department of Health and Human Services. The mission of the VR program is to promote employment and independence for people with disabilities. Its services include counseling, training, education, medical assistance, and transportation to qualified individuals (North Carolina Department of Health and Human Services 2009a).

WIC (Women, Infants, and Children): WIC provides federal grants to states for supplemental foods, health care referrals, and nutrition education for low-income pregnant, breastfeeding, and non-breastfeeding postpartum women and to infants and children up to age five who are found to be at nutritional risk (U.S. Department of Agriculture Food and Nutrition Service 2015).

Notes

1. "Other" Stories

1. Farmer (1996) and Susser (2009) both position the HIV/AIDS epidemic and related structures of care within frameworks of global neoliberalism; however, both fine examples of scholarship take broader macro-level approaches in favor of highlighting inequity as a factor in the global epidemic. As a result neither project examines ethnographic specificities of the American epidemic.

2. The Ryan White CARE Act comprises four major program titles: Title I provides grants to eligible metropolitan areas (EMAs) that have been disproportionately affected by the epidemic. Title II issues grants to the states, the District of Columbia, Puerto Rico, and U.S. territories to improve the delivery of health care and support services for people living with HIV/AIDS. Title III furnishes direct grants to non-profit entities for primary care and early intervention services. Title IV provides grants for family-centered care for infants, children, youth, and women living with HIV disease and their families (Institute of Medicine 2004). In 2006 the program's "titles" were changed to "parts."

3. To be eligible for EMA status (and thus Title I funding), an area must have at least two thousand reported AIDS cases during the previous five years and a total population of at least five hundred thousand.

4. "AIDS Is Now the Leading Killer of Americans from 25–44," *New York Times*, January 31, 1995.

5. Obviously I cannot do justice to the volume of HIV research studies published during this period. Here I offer a strategic few citations that the HRSA has cited in its "official" renderings of the history of the epidemic and in Farmer et al.'s (1996) seminal volume *Women, Poverty, and AIDS: Sex, Drugs, and Structural Violence.*

6. Having a separate line item means that ADAP became a significant service in its own right, requiring a budget based on its own formulary. Title II refers to funding distributed among states.

7. The Congressional Black Caucus is a formal Democratic select committee. At the time of my research it had thirty-eight members; currently it consists of forty-six individuals. It functions to positively influence issues and events pertinent to African Americans. The Minority AIDS Initiative represents the caucus's response to HIV/AIDS.

8. Bourgois (2001) contends that that the culture of poverty concept endured into the 1990s because it fit well with American ideologies of a meritocratic society. The logic of the "open society" concept posited that the socially immobile had only themselves to blame for their limitations or difficult life circumstances.

2. *The Local Landscape*

1. CD4 cells are a type of white blood cell, also known as a CD4+, or t-lymphocyte, cell. The cells that HIV infects are most often CD4 cells. With HIV infection the DNA of the virus becomes part of the CD4 cell. Paradoxically when CD4 cells multiply as an immune response to the infection, they also make more replications of the virus. As the virus progresses, the body makes fewer CD4 cells while copies of the virus proliferate. A person with fewer than two hundred CD4 cells is considered to have AIDS (Centers for Disease Control 1992). A viral load test measures the amount of HIV virus in the blood. Currently tests can detect anywhere from five copies to a million copies per milliliter of blood. Viral load testing along with CD4 cell count testing can provide insight as to the efficacy of drug treatments and disease course (Peter and Sevall 2004).

2. When I returned to the field in May 2009, the new fiscal year had just begun for the Ryan White programs. The new fiscal year ushered in an important change for the provision of Emergency Financial Assistance Programs. Under the new federal guideline, HIV support service clients were eligible for a maximum of twenty-one weeks of emergency financial support. For example, if Health Partnership paid a client's rent one month, then that payment was considered four weeks of support. This change represented the first time that formal and federally mandated restrictions had been placed on emergency financial assistance at Health Partnership.

3. When I returned for follow-up activities, Health Partnership had already begun to participate in the federal program for nutritional assistance, the Emergency Food Assistance Program. Health Partnership received monthly deliveries of fresh, frozen, and canned food. Recipients had to qualify for the "extra" food by proving their financial need and had to receive or at least qualify for food stamps. Not all clients at Health

Partnership could prove this need despite their regular participation in Health Partnership assistance programs and food pantry services.

4. SSDI and SSI both provide monthly benefits checks for disabled persons living with HIV/AIDS. Persons who have worked in the preceding ten years and have paid Social Security taxes are eligible for SSDI. Persons who do not have a consistent work history or who have not paid Social Security taxes are eligible for SSI. In some cases where an individual has very few resources and a history of consistently very low-income employment, they may receive benefits from both programs (Social Security Administration 2009).

5. Recipients of disability insurance benefits can earn up to $979 per month in additional income. Anyone earning $980 or more per month is considered able to participate in "substantial gainful activity" (Social Security Administration 2009).

6. The paper food stamps of decades past were long gone by the time of this study. In Midway women carried an electronic benefits transfer (EBT) card. Each month the Department of Health and Human Services deposited each woman's allotment of food stamp money into her EBT account. Once the money had been transferred to the account, women could use their EBT cards like debit cards. While EBT cards were appreciated as being more discrete than their paper counterparts, they did not allow women to receive cash back for their purchases. EBT cards were officially designed in this way to reduce fraud and the mishandling of federal money for nutritional assistance (North Carolina Division of Social Services 2009).

7. North Carolina officially calculated food stamp benefits based on monthly income and household size. For a single woman with no children, the monthly income limit at the time of this research was $1,127. A woman who received $1,127 each month in income technically qualified for $176 in food stamps (North Carolina Division of Social Services 2009). Many women, however, reported incomes far below the monthly limit and still received less than the maximum benefit allotment. This situation could have resulted from inaccurate paperwork on the part of Social Service employees or inaccurate income reporting on the part of study participants. In some cases the women explained that rent and utilities subsidies affected their benefits calculations, and women in other cases were unsure why they did not receive more food stamps than they did.

8. Health Partnership employees often struggled with the idea of fee-for-service case management. On the one hand, it provided income to the organization. As case manager salaries were paid through United Way

funds and Ryan White funds, Medicaid billing money essentially represented a potential cash flow in the broader organization. Cash flow allowed employees to spend down their budgets more effectively because they could wait longer to be reimbursed by the state's Ryan White consortium. They would also have more disposable monies for agency-sponsored programs and events.

On the other hand, case managers worried that entering into the fee-for-service case management arrangement would cause commotion in the broader community. Employees worried that other organizations would resent Health Partnership because they already received the lion's share of Ryan White Part B funds in the community. In addition, employees worried that clients would expect them to expand the boundaries of their services to informally include transportation.

3. Urban Poverty Three Ways

1. *Boosting* is when a person steals items from businesses and/or homes and then sells them.

4. The Pedagogy of Policy Reform

1. Community Advisory Boards (CABS) came out of the AIDS Clinical Trials Groups of the 1980s that advocated for broader inclusion and the expedient processing and disseminating of the information and results from clinical trials. Their current form emerged in the early 1990s. CAB members tend to be nonscientists who might represent a range of community interests such as schools, religious groups, and/or community-based organizations. CABS conduct outreach, review and evaluate protocol for clinical trials, and facilitate productive relationships between researchers and the broader communities in which they work (AIDS Clinical Trials Group 2015).
2. According to the guest speaker, Selzentry was approved as an "entry inhibitor" in August 2007. Entry inhibitors essentially prevent the HIV virus from attaching to otherwise healthy cells (Briz, Poveda, and Soriano 2006; Dolin 2008; Este and Telenti 2007). Isentress, approved in October 2007, is an integrase inhibitor, which prevents the HIV virus from attaching to DNA molecules once the virus has entered the cell (Evering and Markowitz 2008; Havlir 2008). Approved in January 2008, Intelence is a non-nucleoside reverse transcriptase inhibitor, which prevents HIV replication in the body (DiNubile 2008).
3. Health Partnership was not reimbursed for money spent on a client when the services provided were not properly documented.

5. Using "Survival," Part I

1. The idea of "owning past mistakes" is referred to in the Twelve Steps of Alcoholics Anonymous (2014).

2. A "spend down" is part of budget realignment, or the process of spending federal funds to match the projected budgets submitted to the federal government. Budget realignment happened when the agency had not spent all of the money to which it was entitled. If it did not spend the money, it would receive less funding the following year. Periodically the state HIV/AIDS consortium advised agencies to spend down their funds so that the proposed budgets would match the actual amount of money spent on services and programs.

3. This average refers to self-reported requests during the 2007–8 and 2009 research periods. When I returned in 2012, the support requests by all study participants with whom I remained in contact had dropped off considerably. This decrease was, in part, due to the changes described in chapter 1 and the informal services criterion for eligibility explained in chapter 4.

4. The Black Church Week of Prayer is held every year across the nation. Its goal is to include area churches in the dialogue concerning the HIV epidemic. It is a week of support, education, and community involvement. At the time of this research, HIV/AIDS was still heavily stigmatized in Midway. The stigmatization of HIV disease often meant that the women's illnesses, experiences, and needs were little discussed as a part of the city's "Black mainstream" political, social, and/or economic agenda (see Cohen 1999). Thus institutions in the Black community still often regarded HIV disease as a disease of the "other" or of the "undeserving" (Berger 2004; Jones-DeWeever 2005). This week marked for some women in this study one of the few moments when their church congregations acknowledged the epidemic and the struggles of persons living with HIV.

References

Abu-Lughod, Lila. 1986. *Veiled Sentiments: Honor and Poetry in a Bedouin Society*. Berkeley: University of California Press.

Act Up/NY Women and AIDS Book Group. 1990. *Women, AIDS, and Activism*. Boston: South End Press.

AIDS Clinical Trials Group. 2015. "History of the ACTG." https://actgnetwork .org/History.

Aggleton, Peter, Peter Davies, and Graham Hart, eds. 1997. *AIDS: Activism and Alliances*. Social Aspects of AIDS. London: Taylor & Francis.

Alcabes, P., A. Muñoz, D. Vlahov, and G. H. Friedland. 1993. "Incubation Period of Human Immunodeficiency Virus." *Epidemiologic Reviews* 15 (2): 303–18.

Alcabes, P., E. E. Schoenbaum, and R. S. Klein. 1993. "Correlates of the Rate of Decline of CD4+ Lymphocytes among Injection Drug Users Infected with the Human Immunodeficiency Virus." *American Journal of Epidemiology* 137 (9): 989–1000.

Alcoholics Anonymous. 2014. *Twelve Steps*. http://www.aa.org/pages_enUS /twelve-steps-and-twelve-traditions.

Ameisen, J. C., and A. Capron. 1991. "Cell Dysfunction and Depletion in AIDS: The Programmed Cell Death Hypothesis." *Immunology Today* 12 (4): 102–5.

Bacellar, H., A. Muñoz, D. R. Hoover, J. P. Phair, D. R. Besley, L. A. Kingsley, and S. H. Vermund. 1994. "Incidence of Clinical AIDS Conditions in a Cohort of Homosexual Men with CD4+ Cell Counts < 100/MM3." *Journal of Infectious Diseases* 170 (5): 1284–87.

Baer, Hans, Merrill Singer, and Ida Susser. 1997. *Medical Anthropology and the World System: A Critical Perspective*. Westport CT: Bergin and Garvey.

Barnett, Tony, and Alan Whiteside. 2002. *AIDS in the Twenty-First Century: Disease and Globalization*. New York: Palgrave Macmillan.

Battle, Sheila. 1997. "The Bond Is Called Blackness: Black Women and AIDS." In *The Gender Politics of HIV/AIDS in Women: Perspectives on the Pandemic in the United States*, edited by Nancy Goldstein and Jennifer Manlowe, 282–92. New York: New York University Press.

Becherer, P. R., M. L. Smiley, T. J. Matthews, K. J. Weinhold, C. W. McMillan, and G. C. White. 1990. "Human Immunodeficiency Virus-1 Disease Progression in Hemophiliacs." *American Journal of Hematology* 34 (3): 204–9.

Berger, Michele Tracy. 2004. *Workable Sisterhood: The Political Journey of Stigmatized Women with HIV/AIDS*. Princeton NJ: Princeton University Press.

Biehl, João. 2004. "The Activist State: Global Pharmaceuticals, AIDS, and Citizenship in Brazil." *Social Text* 22 (3): 105–32.

———. 2007. *Will to Live: AIDS Therapies and the Politics of Survival*. Princeton NJ: Princeton University Press.

Bolles, A. Lynn. 2001. "Seeking the Ancestors: Forging a Black Feminist Tradition in Anthropology." In *Black Feminist Anthropology: Theory, Politics, Praxis, and Poetics*, edited by Irma McClaurin, 1–23. New Brunswick NJ: Rutgers University Press.

Booth, Karen. 2004. *Local Women, Global Science: Fighting AIDS in Kenya*. Bloomington: Indiana University Press.

Bourdieu, Pierre. 1986. "The Forms of Capital." In *Handbook of Theory and Research for the Sociology of Education*, edited by J. Richardson, 241–58. New York: Greenwood.

Bourgois, Philippe. 1996. *In Search of Respect: Selling Crack in El Barrio*. New York: Cambridge University Press.

———. 2000. "Disciplining Addictions: The Bio-Politics of Methadone and Heroin in the United States." *Culture, Medicine, and Psychiatry* 24 (2): 165–95.

———. 2001. "Culture of Poverty." In *International Encyclopedia of the Social and Behavioral Sciences*, edited by Neil J. Smelser and Paul B. Baltes, 11904–7. New York: Elsevier.

Bridges, K. M. 2011. *Reproducing Race: An Ethnography of Pregnancy as a Site of Racialization*. Berkeley: University of California Press.

Briz, Veronica, Eva Poveda, and Vincent Soriano. 2006. "HIV Entry Inhibitors: Mechanisms of Action and Resistance Pathways." *Journal of Antimicrobial Chemotherapy* 57 (4): 619–27.

Brodkin, Karen. 2000. "Global Capitalism: What's Race Got to Do with It?" *American Ethnologist* 27 (2): 237–56.

Buchbinder, S. P., M. H. Katz, N. A. Hessol, P. M. O'Malley, and S. D. Holmberg. 1994. "Long-Term HIV-1 Infection without Immunologic Progression." *AIDS* 8 (8): 1123–28.

Buck, Pem Davidson. 1994. "'Arbeit Macht Frei': Racism and Bound, Concentrated Labor in U.S. Prisons." *Urban Anthropology and Studies of Cultural Systems and World Economic Development* 23 (4): 331–72.

Butler, Melba, and Chedgzsey Smith-McKeever. 2003. "Focus on Solutions: Harlem Dowling–West Side Center for Children and Family Services: A Comprehensive Response to Working with HIV-Affected Children and Families." In *African American Women and HIV/AIDS: Critical Responses*, edited by Dorie J. Gilbert and Ednita M. Wright, 101–6. Westport CT: Praeger.

Caldwell, Cleopatra Howard, Barbara J. Guthrie, and James S. Jackson. 2006. "Identity Development, Discrimination, and Psychological Well-being among African American and Caribbean Black Adolescents." In *Gender, Race, Class and Health: Intersectional Approaches*, edited by Amy Schulz and Leith Mullings, 163–91. San Francisco: Jossey-Bass.

Carovano, Kathryn. 1991. "More Than Mothers and Whores: Redefining the Prevention Needs of Women." *International Journal of Health Services* 21 (1): 131–42.

Carr, E. Summerson. 2011. *Scripting Addiction: The Politics of Therapeutic Talk and American Sobriety.* Princeton NJ: Princeton University Press.

Castro, Arachu, and Merrill Singer, eds. 2004. *Unhealthy Health Policy: A Critical Anthropological Examination.* Walnut Creek CA: AltaMira Press.

Centers for Disease Control and Prevention (CDC). 1992. "1993 Revised Classification System for HIV Infection and Expanded Surveillance Case Definition for AIDS among Adolescents and Adults." *Morbidity and Mortality Weekly Report* 41 (RR-17): 1–19.

———. 1993. "Revised Classification System for HIV Infection and Expanded Surveillance Case Definition for AIDS among Adolescents and Adults." *Morbidity and Mortality Weekly Report* 41 (December): 1–19.

———. 1995. "Update: AIDS among Women—United States, 1994." *Morbidity and Mortality Weekly Report* 44 (5): 81–84.

———. 2015. "Health Disparities in HIV/AIDS, Viral Hepatitis, STDs, and TB." July 30. www.cdc.gov/nchhstp/healthdisparities/AfricanAmericans.html.

Chase, Sabrina. 2011. *Surviving HIV/AIDS in the Inner City: How Resourceful Latinas Beat the Odds.* New Brunswick NJ: Rutgers University Press.

Chien, Arnold, Margaret Connors, and Kenneth Fox Jr. 2000. "The Drug War in Perspective." In *Dying for Growth: Global Inequality and the Health of the Poor*, edited by Jim Yong Kim, Joyce V. Millen, Alec Irwin, and John Gershman, 293–330. Monroe ME: Common Courage Press.

Cleage, Pearl. 1997. *What Looks Like Crazy on an Ordinary Day.* New York: Harper.

Coates, R. A., V. T. Farewell, J. Raboud, S. E. Read, D. K. MacFadden, L. M. Calzavara, J. K. Johnson, F. A. Shepherd, and M. M. Fanning. 1990. "Cofactors of Progression to Acquired Immunodeficiency Syndrome in a Cohort of Male Sexual Contacts of Men with Human Immunodeficiency Virus Disease." *American Journal of Epidemiology* 132 (4): 717–22.

Cohen, Cathy J. 1999. *The Boundaries of Blackness: AIDS and the Breakdown of Black Politics*. Chicago: University of Chicago Press.

Collins, Jane. 2008. "The Specter of Slavery: Workfare and the Economic Citizenship of Poor Women." In *New Landscapes of Inequality: Neoliberalism and the Erosion of Democracy in America*, edited by Jane Collins, Micaela di Leonardo, and Brett Williams, 131–52. Santa Fe NM: School for Advanced Research Press.

Collins, Patricia Hill. 1990. *Black Feminist Thought: Knowledge, Consciousness, and the Politics of Empowerment*. Boston: Unwin Hyman.

———. 2001. *Black Sexual Politics: African Americans, Gender, and the New Racism*. New York: Routledge.

Comaroff, J. 2007. "Beyond Bare Life: AIDS (Bio)Politics, and the Neoliberal Order." *Public Culture* 19 (1): 197–219.

Comaroff, J., and J. L. Comaroff. 2001. "Millennial Capitalism: First Thoughts on a Second Coming." In *Millennial Capitalism and the Culture of Neoliberalism*, edited by J. Comaroff and J. L. Comaroff, 1–56. Durham NC: Duke University Press.

Connors, Margaret. 1992. "Risk Perception, Risk Taking, and Risk Management among Intravenous Drug Users: Implications for AIDS Prevention." *Social Science and Medicine* 34 (6): 591–601.

———. 1996. "Sex, Drugs, and Structural Violence: Unraveling the Epidemic among Poor Women of Color in the United States." In *Women, Poverty, and AIDS: Sex, Drugs, and Structural Violence*, edited by Paul Farmer, Margaret Connors, and Janie Simmons, 91–123. Monroe ME: Common Courage Press.

Corbett, K. P. 2009. "'You've Got It, You May Have It, You Haven't Got It': Multiplicity, Heterogeneity, and the Unintended Consequences of HIV-Related Tests." *Science Technology Human Values* 34 (1): 102–25.

Cox, Robert Henry. 1998. "The Consequences of Welfare Reform: How Conceptions of Social Rights Are Changing." *Journal of Social Policy* 27 (1): 1–16.

Crenshaw, Kimberlé. 1989. "Demarginalizing the Intersection of Race and Sex: A Black Feminist Critique of Antidiscrimination Doctrine, Feminist Theory, and Antiracist Politics." *University of Chicago Legal Forum*, 139–67.

Danziger, Sheldon, and Ann Chih Lin, eds. 2000. *Coping with Poverty: The*

Social Contexts of Neighborhood, Work, and Family. Ann Arbor: University of Michigan Press.

Davis, Dana-Ain. 2004. "Manufacturing Mammies: The Burdens of Service Work and Welfare Reform among Battered Women." *Anthropologica* 46 (2): 273–88.

———. 2006. *Battered Black Women and Welfare Reform: Between a Rock and a Hard Place*. Albany: State University of New York Press.

Dickover, R. E., M. Dillon, S. G. Gillette, A. Deveikis, M. Keller, S. Plaeger-Marshall, I. Chen, A. Diagne, E. R. Stiehm, and Y. Bryson. 1994. "Rapid Increases in Load of Human Immunodeficiency Virus Correlate with Early Disease Progression and Loss of CD4 Cells in Vertically Infected Infants." *Journal of Infectious Diseases* 170 (5): 1279–84.

Di Leonardo, Micaela. 1998. *Exotics at Home: Anthropologies, Others, American Modernity*. Chicago: University of Chicago Press.

———. 2008. "Introduction: New Global and American Landscapes of Inequality." In *New Landscapes of Inequality: Neoliberalism and the Erosion of Democracy in America*, edited by Jane L. Collins, Micaela di Leondardo, and Brett Williams, 3–20. Santa Fe NM: School for Advanced Research Press.

DiNubile, Mark J. 2008. "Nonnucleotide Reverse-Transcriptase Inhibitors and Treatment Interruption." *Clinical Infectious Diseases* 47 (12): 1602.

Dolin, Raphael. 2008. "A New Class of Anti-HIV Therapy and New Challenges." *New England Journal of Medicine* 359 (14): 1509–11.

Doyal, Lesley. 1995. *What Makes Women Sick: Gender and the Political Economy of Health*. New Brunswick NJ: Rutgers University Press.

Englund, Harri. 2006. *Prisoners of Freedom: Human Rights and the African Poor*. Berkeley: University of California Press.

Epstein, Steven. 1996. *Impure Science: AIDS, Activism, and the Politics of Knowledge*. Berkeley: University of California Press.

Este, T. A., and A. Telenti. 2007. "HIV Entry Inhibitors." *Lancet* 370 (9581): 81–88.

Evering, Teresa H., and Martin Markowitz. 2008. "HIV-1 Integrase Inhibitors." *Physicians' Research Network* 13: 1–9.

Farmer, Paul. 1996. "Women, Poverty, and AIDS." *In Women, Poverty, and AIDS: Sex, Drugs, and Structural Violence*, edited by Paul Farmer, Margaret Connors, and Janie Simmons, 3–38. Monroe ME: Common Courage Press.

Farmer, Paul, Margaret Connors, and Janie Simmons, eds. 1996. *Women, Poverty, and AIDS: Sex, Drugs, and Structural Violence*. Monroe ME: Common Courage Press.

Federal Emergency Management Agency (FEMA). 2015. *FEMA—Emergency*

Food and Shelter Program Fact Sheet. July 30. http://www.fema.gov
/recovery-directorate/emergency-food-shelter-program-fact-sheet.

Ferguson, James. 2006. *Global Shadows: Africa in the Neoliberal World Order*.
Durham NC: Duke University Press.

Fischl, M. A., D. D. Richman, N. Hansen, A. C. Collier, J. T. Carey, M. F. Para,
W. D. Hardy, et al. 1990. "The Safety and Efficacy of Zidovudine (AZT) in
the Treatment of Subjects with Mildly Symptomatic Human Immunodeficiency Virus Type I (HIV) Infection: A Double-Blind, Placebo-Controlled
Trial." *Annals of Internal Medicine* 112 (10): 727–37.

Foley, Ellen E. 2009. *Your Pocket Is What Cures You: The Politics of Health in
Senegal*. New Brunswick NJ: Rutgers University Press.

Food Bank of Central and Eastern North Carolina. 2012–13. "Frequently Asked
Questions." http://www.foodbankcenc.org/site/PageServer?pagename
=hunger–faqs#oget.

Foucault, Michel. 1978. *The History of Sexuality*. Vol. 1, *An Introduction*. New
York: Vintage Books.

Freire, Paulo. [1970] 2000. *Pedagogy of the Oppressed*. Translated by Myra
Bergman Ramos. New York: Bloomsbury Academic.

Friedland, Gerald H., Brian Saltzman, Joan Vileno, Katherine Freeman, Lewis
K. Schrager, and Robert S. Klein. 1991. "Survival Differences in Patients
with AIDS." *Journal of Acquired Immune Deficiency Syndromes* 4 (2):
144–53.

Fullilove, Mindy Thompson, Robert E. Fullilove III, Katherine Haynes, and
Shirley Gross. 1990. "Black Women and AIDS Prevention: A View towards
Understanding the Gender Rules." *Journal of Sex Research* 27 (1): 47–64.

Fullilove, Robert E. 2006. *African Americans, Health Disparities and HIV/AIDS:
Recommendations for Confronting the Epidemic in Black America*. Washington DC: National Minority AIDS Council. http://www.weourselves.org
/reports/NMAC_final_report.pdf.

Galster, George, Ronald Mincy, and Mitchell Tobin. 2004. "The Disparate
Racial Neighborhood Impacts of Metropolitan Economic Restructuring."
In *Race, Poverty, and Domestic Policy*, edited by Michael Henry, 188–218.
New Haven CT: Yale University Press.

Geertz, Clifford. [1973] 2000. *The Interpretation of Cultures*. New York: Basic
Books.

Gilks, C. F., S. Crowley, R. Ekpini, S. Gove, J. Perriens, Y. Souteyrand, D.
Sutherland, M. Vitoria, T. Guerma, and K. De Cock. 2006. "The WHO
Public-Health Approach to Antiretroviral Treatment against HIV in
Resource-Limited Settings." *Lancet* 368 (9534): 505–10.

Goldstein, Donna M. 2001. "Microenterprise Training Programs, Neoliberal

Common Sense, and the Discourses of Self-Esteem." In *The New Poverty Studies: The Ethnography of Power, Politics, and Impoverished People in the United States*, edited by Judith Goode and Jeff Maskovsky, 236–72. New York: New York University Press.

Goldstein, Nancy. 1997. Introduction. In *The Gender Politics of HIV/AIDS in Women: Perspectives on the Pandemic in the United States*, edited by Nancy Goldstein and Jennifer Manlowe, 1–24. New York: New York University Press.

Gollub, Erica L. 1999. "Human Rights Is a U.S. Problem, Too: The Case of Women and HIV." *American Journal of Public Health* 89 (10): 1479–82.

Goode, Judith. 2002a. "From New Deal to Bad Deal: Racial and Political Implications of U.S. Welfare Reform." In *Western Welfare in Decline: Globalization and Women's Poverty*, edited by Catherine Kingfisher, 65–89. Philadelphia: University of Pennsylvania Press.

———. 2002b. "How Urban Ethnography Counters Myths about the Poor." In *Urban Life: Readings in the Anthropology of the City*, edited by George Gmelch, Robert V. Kemper, and Walter P. Zenner. 185–201. Long Grove IL: Waveland Press.

Goode, Judith, and Jeff Maskovsky, eds. 2001. *The New Poverty Studies: The Ethnography of Power, Politics, and Impoverished People in the United States*. New York: New York University Press.

Gould, Deborah B. 2009. *Moving Politics: Emotion and ACT UP's Fight against AIDS*. Chicago: University of Chicago Press.

Graham, N. M., S. L. Zeger, L. P. Park, S. H. Vermund, R. Detels, C. R. Rinaldo, and J. P. Phair. 1992. "The Effects on Survival of Early Treatment of Human Immunodeficiency Virus Infection." *New England Journal of Medicine* 326 (16): 1037–42.

Guell, Cornelia. 2011. "Candi(e)d Action: Biosocialities of Turkish Berliners Living with Diabetes." *Medical Anthropology Quarterly* 25 (3): 377–94.

Harrington, Michael. 1962. *The Other America: Poverty in the United States*. New York: Scribner.

Harvey, David. 2005. *A Brief History of Neoliberalism*. New York: Oxford University Press.

Havlir, Diane V. 2008. "HIV Integrase Inhibitors—out of the Pipeline and into the Clinic." *New England Journal of Medicine* 359 (4): 416–18.

Hays, S. 2003. *Flat Broke with Children: Women in the Age of Welfare Reform*. New York: Oxford University Press.

Health Resources and Services Administration (HRSA). 2001. *A Primer on Title I and Title II Formula Allocation Calculations*. Unpublished document.

———. 2010. *Going the Distance: The Ryan White HIV/AIDS Program—20 Years of Leadership, a Legacy of Care*. Rockville MD: Health Resources and Services Administration.

———. 2014a. *A Living History: The Ryan White HIV/AIDS Program*. June 12. http://Hab.hrsa.gov/livinghistory/index.htm.

———. 2014b. "Program Guidance: Priority Setting and Resource Allocation." In *Ryan White HIV/AIDS Program Part A Manual*. June 16. http://hab.hrsa.gov/tools2/PartA/parta/ptAsec7chap2.htm.

Henrici, Jane. 2002. "U.S. Women and Poverty." *Voices* 6 (1): 27–31.

Henry, C. Michael. 2004. "Introduction: Historical Overview of Race and Poverty from Reconstruction to 1969." In *Race, Poverty, and Domestic Policy*, edited by C. Michael Henry, 1–56. New Haven CT: Yale University Press.

Hill, Benjamin. 1991. "Solomon Fry, Survivor." *Anthropology and Humanism Quarterly* 16 (4): 120–28.

Hochschild, A. 2003. *The Managed Heart: The Commercialization of Human Feeling*. Twentieth anniversary ed. Berkeley: University of California Press.

Horton, Sarah. 2006. "The Double Burden on Safety Net Providers: Placing Health Disparities in the Context of the Privatization of Health Care in the United States." *Social Science & Medicine* 63 (10): 2702–14.

Horton, Sarah, and Judith C. Barker. 2009. "'Stains' on their Self-Discipline: Public Health, Hygiene, and the Disciplining of Undocumented Immigrant Parents in the Nation's Internal Borderlands." *American Ethnologist* 36 (4): 784–98.

Institute of Medicine. 2004. *Measuring What Matters: Allocation, Planning, and Quality Assessment for the Ryan White CARE Act*. Washington DC: National Academies Press.

Jing, Shao L. 2006. "Fluid Labor and Blood Money: The Economy of HIV/AIDS in Rural Central China." *Cultural Anthropology* 21 (4): 535–69.

Jones-DeWeever, Avis A. 2005. "Saving Ourselves: African American Women and the HIV/AIDS Crisis." *Harvard Journal of African American Public Policy* 11: 79–83.

Kaiser Family Foundation. 2006. *State Health Facts*. September 26. http://kff.org/statedata.

Kalofonos, I. A. 2010. "'All I Eat Is ARVs': The Paradox of AIDS Treatment Interventions in Central Mozambique." *Medical Anthropology Quarterly* 24 (3): 363–80.

Katz, M. H., L. Hsu, M. Lingo, G. Woelffer, and S. K. Schwarcz. 1998. "Impact of Socioeconomic Status on Survival with AIDS." *American Journal of Epidemiology* 148 (3): 282–91.

Keating, Peter, and Alberto Cambrioso. 2003. *Biomedical Platforms: Realign-*

ing the Normal and the Pathological in Late-Twentieth-Century Medicine. Cambridge MA: MIT Press.

Keet, I. P., A. Krol, M. R. Klein, P. Veugelers, J. de Wit, M. Roos, M. Koot, J. Goudsmit, F. Miedema, and R. A. Coutinho. 1994. "Characteristics of Long-Term Asymptomatic Infection with Human Immunodeficiency Virus Type I in Men with Normal and Low CD4+ Cell Counts." *Journal of Infectious Diseases* 169 (6): 1236–43.

Kim, Jim Yong, Joyce V. Millen, Alec Irwin, and John Gershman, eds. 2000. *Dying for Growth: Global Inequality and the Health of the Poor*. Monroe ME: Common Courage Press.

Kingfisher, Catherine. 2001. "Producing Disunity: The Constraints and Incitements of Welfare Work." In *The New Poverty Studies: The Ethnography of Power, Politics, and Impoverished People in the United States*, edited by Judith Goode and Jeff Maskovsky, 273–92. New York: New York University Press.

———. 2002. "Neoliberalism I: Discourses of Personhood and Welfare Reform." In *Western Welfare in Decline: Globalization and Women's Poverty*, edited by Catherine Kingfisher, 13–31. Philadelphia: University of Pennsylvania Press.

Kingfisher, Catherine, and Michael Goldsmith. 2001. "Reforming Women in the United States and Aotearoa/New Zealand: A Comparative Ethnography of Welfare Reform in Global Context." *American Anthropologist* 103 (3): 714–32.

Koblin, B. A., P. E. Taylor, P. Rubinstein, and C. E. Stevens. 1992. "Effect of Zidovudine on Survival in HIV-I Infection: Observational Data from a Cohort Study of Gay Men." Paper presented at Eighth International Conference on AIDS, July 19–24, Amsterdam, abstract no. PoC 4349.

Koenig, S. P., F. Leondre, and P. Farmer. 2004. "Scaling-Up HIV Treatment Programmes in Resource-Limited Settings: The Rural Haiti Experience." *AIDS* 18 (no. S3): S21–S25.

Koester, Stephen, and Judith Schwartz. 1993. "Crack, Gangs, Sex, and Powerlessness: A View from Denver." In *Crack Pipe as Pimp: An Ethnographic Investigation of Sex-for-Crack Exchanges*, edited by Mitchell S. Ratner, 187–204. New York: Lexington Books.

Lane, Sandra D., Robert A. Rubinstein, Robert H. Keefe, Noah Webster, Donald A. Cibula, Alan Rosenthal, and Jesse Dowdell. 2004. "Structural Violence and Racial Disparity in HIV Transmission." *Journal of Health Care for the Poor and Underserved* 15 (3): 319–35.

Leacock, Eleanor Burke, ed. 1971. *The Culture of Poverty: A Critique*. New York: Simon & Schuster.

Lehman, Jeffrey, and Sheldon Danziger. 2004. "Turning Our Backs on the New Deal: The End of Welfare in 1996." In *Race, Poverty, and Domestic Policy*, edited by C. Michael Henry, 603–30. New Haven CT: Yale University Press.

Lemp, G. F., A. M. Hirozawa, D. Givertz, G. N. Nieri, L. Anderson, M. L. Lindegren, R. S. Janssen, and M. Katz. 1994. "Seroprevalence of HIV and Risk Behaviors among Young Homosexual and Bisexual Men: The San Francisco/Berkeley Young Men's Survey." *Journal of the American Medical Association* 272 (6): 449–54.

Levine, Robert S., Nathaniel C. Briggs, Barbara S. Kilbourne, William D. King, Yvonne Fry-Johnson, Peter T. Baltrus, Baqar A. Husaini, and George S. Rust. 2007. "Black-White Mortality from HIV in the United States before and after Introduction of Highly Active Antiretroviral Therapy in 1996." *American Journal of Public Health* 97 (10): 1884–92.

Lewis, Oscar. 1959. *Five Families: Mexican Case Studies in the Culture of Poverty*. New York: Basic Books.

Lipsky, Michael. 1980. *Street-Level Bureaucracy: Dilemmas of the Individual in Public Services*. New York: Russell Sage Foundation.

Marsland, Rebecca. 2012. "(Bio)sociality and HIV in Tanzania: Finding a Living to Support a Life." *Medical Anthropology Quarterly* 26 (4): 470–85.

Marsland, Rebecca, and Ruth Prince. 2012. "What Is Life Worth? Exploring Biomedical Interventions, Survival, and the Politics of Life." *Medical Anthropology Quarterly* 26 (4): 453–69.

Martin, Emily. 1994. *Flexible Bodies: Tracking Immunity in American Culture from the Days of Polio to the Age of AIDS*. New York: Beacon Press.

———. 2012. "Grafting Together Medical Anthropology, Feminism, and Technoscience." In *Medical Anthropology at the Intersections: Histories, Activisms, and Futures*, edited by Marcia C. Inhorn and Emily A. Wentzell, 23–40. Durham NC: Duke University Press.

Marx, R., M. H. Katz, M. S. Park, and R. J. Gurley. 1997. "Meeting the Service Needs of HIV-Infected Persons: Is the Ryan White CARE Act Succeeding?" *Journal of Acquired Immune Deficiency Syndromes and Human Retrovirology* 14 (1): 44–55.

Maskovsky, Jeff. 2000. "'Managing' the Poor: Neoliberalism, Medicaid HMOs, and the Triumph of Consumerism among the Poor." *Medical Anthropology* 19 (2): 121–46.

Maternowska, M. Catherine. 2006. *Reproducing Inequities: Poverty and the Politics of Population in Haiti*. New Brunswick NJ: Rutgers University Press.

McClaurin, Irma, ed. 2001. *Black Feminist Anthropology: Theory, Politics, Praxis, and Poetics*. New Brunswick NJ: Rutgers University Press.

McFarland, W., S. Chen, L. Hsu, S. Schwarcz, and M. Katz. 2003. "Low

Socioeconomic Status Is Associated with a Higher Rate of Death in the Era of Highly Active Antiretroviral Therapy, San Francisco." *Journal of Acquired Immune Deficiency Syndromes* 33 (1): 96–103.

Mohanty, Chandra Talpade. 1991. "Under Western Eyes: Feminist Scholarship and Colonial Discourses." In *Third World Women and the Politics of Feminism*, edited by Chandra Talpade Mohanty, Ann Russo, and Lourdes Torres, 51–80. Bloomington: Indiana University Press.

Moore, Alison, Christopher N. Candlin, and Guenter A. Plum. 2001. "Making Sense of HIV-Related Viral Load: One Expert or Two?" *Culture, Health, and Sexuality* 3 (4): 429–50.

Morgen, Sandra. 2002. *Into Our Own Hands: The Women's Health Movement in the United States, 1969–1990*. New Brunswick NJ: Rutgers University Press.

Morgen, Sandra, and Jeff Maskovsky. 2003. "The Anthropology of Welfare 'Reform': New Perspectives on U.S. Urban Poverty in the Post-Welfare Era." *Annual Review of Anthropology* 32: 315–38.

Morgen, Sandra, and Jill Weigt. 2001. "Poor Women, Fair Work, and Welfare-to-Work." In *The New Poverty Studies: The Ethnography of Power, Politics, and Impoverished People in the United States*, edited by Judith Goode and Jeff Maskovsky, 152–78. New York: New York University Press.

Morgen, Sandra, Joan Acker, and Jill Weigt. 2010. *Stretched Thin: Poor Families, Welfare Work, and Welfare Reform*. Ithaca NY: Cornell University Press.

Morsy, Soheir A. 1993. *Gender, Sickness, and Healing in Rural Egypt: Ethnography in Historical Context*. Boulder CO: Westview Press.

———. 1996. "Political Economy in Medical Anthropology." In *Medical Anthropology: Contemporary Theory and Method*, edited by Carolyn F. Sargent and Thomas M. Johnson, 21–40. Westport CT: Praeger.

Mullings, Leith. 2001. "Households Headed by Women: The Politics of Race, Class, and Gender." In *The New Poverty Studies: The Ethnography of Power, Politics, and Impoverished People in the United States*, edited by Judith Goode and Jeff Maskovsky, 37–56. New York: New York University Press.

———. 2005a. "Interrogating Racism: Toward an Antiracist Anthropology." *Annual Review of Anthropology* 34 (1): 667–93.

———. 2005b. "Resistance and Resilience: The Sojourner Syndrome and the Social Context of Reproduction in Central Harlem." *Transforming Anthropology* 13 (2): 79–91.

Mullings, Leith, and Amy J. Schulz. 2005. "Intersectionality and Health: An Introduction." In *Gender, Race, Class, and Health: Intersectional Approaches*, edited by Amy J. Schulz and Leith Mullings, 3–20. San Francisco: John Wiley and Sons.

Naples, Nancy A. 1998. *Grassroots Warriors: Activist Mothering, Community Work, and the War on Poverty*. New York: Routledge.

National Health Policy Forum. 2010. *The Basics: The Ryan White HIV/AIDS Program*. Washington DC: George Washington University. www.nhpf.org /library/the-basics/Basics_RyanWhite_03-10-10.pdf.

Navarro, Vincente. 2004. "The Politics of Health Inequalities Research in the United States." *International Journal of Health Services* 34 (1): 87–99.

Newman, Katherine. 1994. "Deindustrialization, Poverty, and Downward Mobility: Toward an Anthropology of Economic Disorder." In *Diagnosing America: Anthropology and Public Engagement*, edited by S. Forman, 121–48. Ann Arbor: University of Michigan Press.

———. 2001. "Hard Times on 125th Street: Harlem's Poor Confront Welfare Reform." *American Anthropologist* 103 (3): 762–78.

Nguyen, Vinh-Kim. 2010. *The Republic of Therapy: Triage and Sovereignty in West Africa's Time of AIDS*. Durham NC: Duke University Press.

Nguyen, Vinh-Kim, Cyriaque Yako Ako, Pascal Niamba, Aliou Sylla, and Issoufou Tiendrébéogo. 2007. "Adherence as Therapeutic Citizenship: Impact of the History of Access to Antiretroviral Drugs on Adherence to Treatment." *AIDS* 21 (no. S5): S31–S35.

North Carolina Department of Health and Human Services. 2009a. *Division of Vocational Rehabilitation*. http://www.ncdhhs.gov.dvrs/.

———. 2009b. *Fact Sheet: The North Carolina AIDS Drug Assistance/HIV Medication Program (ADAP)*. http://pdfdrug.com/e/epi.ncpublichealth.com1.html.

North Carolina Division of Social Services. 2009. *Food and Nutrition Services*. November 20. http://www.ncdhhs.gov/dss/foodstamp/index.htm.

North Carolina Rural Center. 2009. *Statewide Labor Markets and Manufacturing Decline*. April 8. www.ncruralcenter.org/index.php?option=com _wrapper&view=wrapper&Itemid=121.

O'Daniel, Alyson. 2009. "Pushing Poverty to the Periphery: HIV-Positive African American Women's Health Needs, the Ryan White CARE Act, and a Political Economy of Service Provision." *Transforming Anthropology* 16 (2): 112–27.

———. 2011. "Access to Medical Care Is Not the Problem: Low-Income Status and Health Care Needs among HIV-Positive African-American Women in Urban North Carolina." *Human Organization* 70 (4): 416–26.

Office of the Press Secretary. The President George W. Bush White House. 2006. *Fact Sheet: The Ryan White HIV/AIDS Treatment Modernization Act of 2006*. December 19. http://georgewbush-whitehouse.archives.gov/news /releases/2006/12/20061219-4.html.

O'Manique, C. 2004. *Neoliberalism and AIDS Crisis in Sub-Saharan Africa: Globalization's Pandemic*. Basingstoke, UK: Palgrave Macmillan.

Ong, Aihwa. 1995. "Making the Biopolitical Subject: Cambodian Immigrants, Refugee Medicine and Cultural Citizenship in California." *Social Science and Medicine* 40 (9): 1243–57.

Palmer, John Logan, and Isabel V. Sawhill, eds. 1982. *The Reagan Experiment*. Washington DC: Urban Institute.

Parada, Jorge P. 2000. "The Changing Face of AIDS." *Minority Health Today* 1 (5): 9–17.

Patillo-McCoy, Mary. 2000. *Black Picket Fences: Privilege and Peril among the Black Middle Class*. Chicago: University of Chicago Press.

People with AIDS Advisory Committee. 1983. *The Denver Principles*. www .actupny.org/documents/denver_principles.pdf.

Peter, J. B., and J. S. Sevall. 2004. "Molecular-Based Methods for Quantifying HIV Viral Load." *AIDS Patient Care and STDs* 18 (2): 75–79.

Petryna, Adriana. 2002. *Life Exposed: Biological Citizens after Chernobyl*. Princeton NJ: Princeton University Press.

Piven, Frances Fox. 1998. "Welfare Reform and the Economic and Cultural Construction of Low Wage Labor Markets." *City and Society* 10 (1): 21–36.
———. 2001. "Welfare Reform and the Economic and Cultural Reconstruction of Low Wage Labor Markets." In *The New Poverty Studies: The Ethnography of Power, Politics, and Impoverished People in the United States*, edited by Judith Goode and Jeff Maskovsky, 135–51. New York: New York University Press.

Pivnick, Anitra, Audrey Jacobson, Kathleen Eric, Lynda Doll, and Ernest Drucker. 1994. "AIDS, HIV Infection and Illicit Drug Use within Inner-City Families and Social Networks." *American Journal of Public Health* 84 (2): 271–74.

Prasad, Monica. 2006. *The Politics of Free Markets: The Rise of Neoliberal Economic Policies in Britain, France, Germany, and the United States*. Chicago: University of Chicago Press.

Quadagno, Jill. 1994. *The Color of Welfare: How Racism Undermined the War on Poverty*. New York: Oxford University Press.

Reese, Ellen. 2005. *Backlash against Welfare Mothers: Past + Present*. Berkeley: University of California Press.

Remien, R. H., A. E. Hirky, M. O. Johnson, L. S. Weinhardt, D. Whittier, and G. M. Le. 2003. "Adherence to Medication Treatment: A Qualitative Study of Facilitators and Barriers among a Diverse Sample of HIV+ Men and Women in Four U.S. Cities." *AIDS and Behavior* 7 (1): 61–72.

Richland, Justin B. 2009. "On Neoliberalism and Other Social Diseases: The

2008 Sociocultural Anthropology Year in Review." *American Anthropologist* 110 (2): 170–76.

Robben, Antonius C. G. M., and Carolyn Nordstrom. 1995. "The Anthropology and Ethnography of Violence and Sociopolitical Conflict." In *Fieldwork under Fire: Contemporary Studies of Violence and Survival*, edited by Carolyn Nordstrom and Antonius C. G. M. Robben, 1–24. Berkeley: University of California Press.

Roberts, Dorothy. 1997. *Killing the Black Body: Race, Reproduction, and the Meaning of Liberty*. New York: Vintage Books.

Rodriguez, Bill. 1997. "Biomedical Models of HIV and Women." In *The Gender Politics of HIV/AIDS in Women: Perspectives on the Pandemic in the United States*, edited by Nancy Goldstein and Jennifer Manlowe, 25–42. New York: New York University Press.

Rose, N., and C. Novas. 2005. "Biological Citizenship." In *Global Assemblages: Technology, Politics, and Ethics as Anthropological Problems*, edited by A. Ong and S. Collier, 439–63. Malden MA: Blackwell.

Rothenberg, Richard, Mary Woelfel, Rand Stoneburner, J. Milberg, R. Parker, and B. Truman. 1987. "Survival with Acquired Immune Deficiency Syndrome: Experience with 5833 Cases in New York City." *New England Journal of Medicine* 317 (21): 1297–302.

Ryan, William. 1976. *Blaming the Victim*. Rev. ed. New York: Vintage Books.

Rylko-Bauer, Barbara, and Paul Farmer. 2002. "Managed Care or Managed Inequality? A Call for Critiques of Market-Based Medicine." *Medical Anthropology Quarterly* 16 (4): 476–502.

Sassen, Saskia. 1996. "Service Employment Regimes and the New Inequality." In *Urban Poverty and the Underclass: A Reader*, edited by Enzo Mingione, 64–82. Cambridge MA: Blackwell.

Scheper-Hughes, Nancy, and Philippe Bourgois, eds. 2003. *Violence in War and Peace: An Anthology*. Malden MA: Blackwell.

Schiller, Nina Glick. 1993. "The Invisible Women: Caregiving and the Construction of AIDS Health Services." *Culture, Medicine, and Psychiatry* 17 (4): 487–512.

Seccombe, Karen. 1998. *"So You Think I Drive a Cadillac?" Welfare Recipients' Perspectives on the System and Its Reform*. Upper Saddle River NJ: Prentice Hall.

Selik, R. M., S. Y. Chu, and J. W. Buehler. 1993. "HIV Infection as Leading Cause of Death among Hispanics in the United States." *American Journal of Public Health* 79 (7): 836–39.

Shilts, Randy. 1987. *And the Band Played On: Politics, People, and the AIDS Epidemic*. New York: St. Martin's Press.

Singer, Merrill. 1991. "Confronting the AIDS Epidemic among IV Drug Users: Does Ethnic Culture Matter?" *AIDS Education and Prevention* 3 (3): 258–83.

———. 1993. "AIDS and the Crisis of the U.S. Urban Poor: The Perspective of Critical Medical Anthropology." *Social Science and Medicine* 39 (7): 931–48.

Singer, Merrill, and Arachu Castro. 2004. "Introduction: Anthropology and Health Policy: A Critical Perspective." In *Unhealthy Health Policy: A Critical Anthropological Examination*, edited by Arachu Castro and Merrill Singer, xi–xix. Walnut Creek CA: AltaMira Press.

Sobo, E. J. 1999. "Love, Jealousy, and Unsafe Sex among Inner-City Women." In *The Political Economy of AIDS* (Critical Approaches in the Health Social Sciences), edited by Merrill Singer, 75–104. Amityville NY: Baywood Publishers.

Social Security Administration. 2009. *2009 Red Book: Overview of Our Disability Programs*. November 25.

Sontag, Susan. 1990. *Illness as Metaphor and AIDS and Its Metaphors*. New York: Farrar, Straus and Giroux.

Speretta, Tommaso, and Loring McAlpin. 2014. *Rebels Rebel: AIDS, Art, and Activism in New York, 1979–1989*. Ghent, Belgium: ASAMER Publishers.

Stack, Carol. 1974. *All Our Kin: Strategies for Survival in a Black Community*. New York: Basic Books.

———. 1996. *Call to Home: African Americans Reclaim the Rural South*. New York: Harper Collins.

Sterk, Claire E. 1999. *Tricking and Tripping: Prostitution in the Era of AIDS*. Putnam Valley NY: Social Change Press.

Stoez, David, and Howard Jacob Karger. 1990. "Welfare Reform: From Illusion to Reality." *Social Work*, March, 141–47.

Stoller, Nancy E. 1998. *Lessons from the Damned: Queers, Whores, and Junkies Respond to AIDS*. New York: Routledge Press.

Stoskopf, Carleen H., Donna L. Richter, and Yang M. Kim. 2001. "Factors Affecting Health Status in African Americans Living with HIV/AIDS." *AIDS Patient Care and STDs* 15 (6): 331–38.

Stover, J., S. Bertozzi, J. P. Gutierrez, N. Walker, K. A. Stanecki, R. Greener, E. Gouws, et al. 2006. "The Global Impact of Scaling Up HIV/AIDS Prevention Programs in Low- and Middle-Income Countries." *Science* 311 (5766): 1474–76.

Susser, Ida. 2009. *AIDS, Sex, and Culture: Global Politics and Survival in Southern Africa*. Oxford, UK: Blackwell.

Tourigny, Sylvie. 1998. "Some New Dying Trick: African American Youth 'Choosing' HIV/AIDS." *Qualitative Health Research* 8 (2): 149–67.

Treichler, Paula. 1999. *How to Have Theory in an Epidemic: Cultural Chronicles of AIDS.* Durham NC: Duke University Press.

Turner, Barbara J., Leona E. Markson, Linda J. McKee, R. Houchens, and T. Fanning. 1994. "Health Care Delivery, Zidovudine Use, and Survival of Women and Men with AIDS." *Journal of Acquired Immune Deficiency Syndromes* 7 (12): 1250–62.

UNAIDS and World Health Organization. 2006. *AIDS Epidemic Update: December 2006.* Geneva, Switzerland: UNAIDS. http://www.who.int/hiv /pub/epidemiology/epiupdate2006/en/.

U.S. Census Bureau. 2011. "What Is AFDC?" October 31. https://www.census .gov/population/socdemo/statbriefs/whatAFDC.html.

U.S. Congress, House of Representatives Committee on Commerce. 2000. *Report on Ryan White CARE Act Amendments of 2000 (106–788).* 106th Cong., 2nd sess., July 25. Lexington KY: BiblioGov Project.

U.S. Department of Agriculture Food and Nutrition Service. 2015. "Women, Infants, and Children (WIC)." www.fns.usda.gov/wic/women-infants-and -children-wic.

U.S. Department of Health and Human Services (USDHHS). 2009a. *About TANF.* December 7. www.acf.hhs.gov/programs/ofa/programs/tanf/about.

———. 2009b. *The HIV/AIDS Program: Legislation.* November 2. www.hab .hrsa.gov/abouthab/legislation.htm.

———. 2009c. *The HIV/AIDS Programs: Caring for the Underserved.* December 3. www.hab.hrsa.gov/about/organization/bureaus/hab/.

———. 2009d. *The Personal Responsibility and Work Opportunity Reconciliation Act of 1996.* http://www.acf.hhs.gov/programs/css/resource/the -personal-responsibility-and-work-opportunity-reconcilliation-act.

———. 2014. "Ryan White HIV/AIDS Program Population Fact Sheet: African Americans." December. http://hab.hrsa.gov/abouthab/populations /africanamericansfs12.pdf.

U.S. Department of Housing and Urban Development. 2009. *Housing Opportunities for People with AIDS.* December 3. www.hud.gov/offices/cpd /aidshousing/programs.

Valverde, E., C. Del Rio, L. Metsch, P. Anderson-Mahoney, C. S. Krawczyk, L. Gooden, and L. I. Gardner. 2004. "Characteristics of Ryan White and Non–Ryan White Funded HIV Medical Care Facilities across Four Metropolitan Areas: Results from the Antiretroviral Treatment and Access Studies Site Survey." *AIDS Care* 16 (7): 841–50.

Ward, Martha C. 1993. "A Different Disease: HIV/AIDS Health Care for Women in Poverty." *Culture, Medicine, and Psychiatry* 17 (4): 413–40.

Waterston, Alisse. 1997. "Anthropological Research and the Politics of HIV

Prevention: Towards a Critique of Policy and Priorities in the Age of AIDS."
Social Science and Medicine 44 (9): 1381–91.

Weber, Lynn. 2006. "Reconstructing the Landscape of Health Disparities
Research: Promoting Dialogue and Collaboration between Feminist
Intersectional and Biomedical Paradigms." In *Gender, Race, Class and
Health: Intersectional Approaches*, edited by Amy Schulz and Leith
Mullings, 21–59. San Francisco: Jossey-Bass.

Whitehead, Tony L. 1997. "Urban Low-Income African American Men, HIV/
AIDS, and Gender Identity." *Medical Anthropology Quarterly* 11 (4): 411–47.

Williams, Sharon E. 2003. "HIV-Positive African American Women and Their
Families: Barriers to Effective Family Coping." In *African American Women
and HIV/AIDS: Critical Responses*, edited by Dorie J. Gilbert and Ednita M.
Wright, 29–50. Westport CT: Praeger.

Wojcicki, J. M. 2002. "'She Drank His Money': Survival Sex and the Problem
of Violence in Taverns in Guateng Province, South Africa." *Medical
Anthropology Quarterly* 16 (3): 267–93.

Wood, E., J. S. Montaner, K. Chan, M. W. Tyndall, M. T. Schechter, D.
Bangsberg, M. V. O'Shaughnessy, and R. S. Hogg. 2002. "Socioeconomic
Status, Access to Triple Therapy, and Survival from HIV Disease since
1996." *AIDS* 16 (15): 2065–72.

World Health Organization. 2015. "Trade, Foreign Policy, Diplomacy, and
Health: Neo-Liberal Ideas." March 22. Who.int/trade/glossary/story067
/en/.

Worth, Dooley. 1989. "Sexual Decision Making and AIDS: Why Condom
Promotion among Vulnerable Women Is Likely to Fail." *Studies in Family
Planning* 20 (6): 297–307.

Young, Steven R., Richard Conviser, Katherine Marconi, and Melanie K.
Wieland. 2003. "Trends and Responsiveness in National Resource
Allocation for Needed HIV Services: A Five Year (1996–2000) Analysis."
Journal of Health and Social Policy 17 (4): 1–4. DOI 10.1300/J045v17n04_01.

Zambrana, Ruth E., and Bonnie Thornton Dill. 2006. "Disparities in Latina
Health: An Intersectional Analysis." In *Gender, Race, Class, and Health:
Intersectional Approaches*, edited by Amy Schulz and Leith Mullings,
192–227. San Francisco: Jossey-Bass.

Index

boosting, 208n1
Bourdieu, Pierre, 131–32
Bourgois, Philippe, 206n8
breathing difficulties, 94, 102
budgets: realignment of, 209n2; spend-down of, 55, 138–39, 143, 155, 207n8, 209n2; and spending freezes, 56, 139, 140
bureaucracy, familiarity with, 131
Bush, George H. W., 26

care providers, 21; Alyson O'Daniel's interactions with, 16–17; boundaries of, 53, 62; client appreciation of, 138, 152; and clients, 76–77, 145, 155; clients' social capital with, 131–62; credentials of, 52–53; criticism of payee role by, 156–57; demographics of, 52; discipline of, by TMA policy, 126–27; and "entitled" clients, 126, 145–48, 189; fund disbursement strategies of, 55–56, 59; interviews with, 13; motivation of, for work, 54; neoliberal worldview of, 75–76, 131, 146, 182, 188; power and powerlessness of, 7, 117–18, 126–27, 132; professionalization of, 52–53; and relaxing of rules, 140, 150; self-disclosure as strategy of, 61; shaming of clients by, 57; stereotyping of clients by, 75–76; "strengths perspective" of, 53–54; styles of, 50–51, 62, 63; survival defined by, 6
CAREWare, 118–20
Carr, E. Summerson: *Scripting Addiction*, 135
Carter, Jimmy, 35
case management: and abusive case

managers, 156–57, 158–59; and case managers' roles, 63, 73, 156–57; fee-for-service, 72, 207n8; Medicaid, 72; medical, 58; nonmedical, 62–64; physical assistance and, 157
CD4 cells, 32–33, 206n1
Chantelle, 60–61, 80–83, 157–58, 177, 178, 180
Charlotte, 106–9, 112, 140, 170, 185
Chase, Sabrina, 77–78, 131
children: and child support, 202; custody struggles for, 84–85, 176; safety of, 108
church, HIV acknowledgment at, 151–52, 209n4
civil rights, White backlash against, 36
Cleage, Pearl: *What Crazy Looks Like on an Ordinary Day*, 33
clients: Alyson O'Daniel as intermediary for, 16–17; banning of, from Health Partnership, 161; care providers' respect for, 50–51, 145; courage of, 130; distancing of, from other clients, 133, 136–37, 138–40, 160–61; empowerment of, 63–64, 123, 142, 168; humanization of, 76–77; "lost to care," 14; and misuse of services, 138, 139, 145–46, 155, 160; and past actions, 85; personal perspectives of, 14–15; privacy of, 48–49; social differences between, 7, 21–22, 77–80, 128, 161–62, 188, 190–91; stereotype of, 10, 75–76, 122, 134, 136–37, 145; survival defined by, 6; and violence, 12; volunteerism of, 109, 140–43, 151–53, 161. *See also* precariously situated women; stable women; vulnerable women

Health Partnership, 47–74; appearance of, 49; banning of clients by, 161; changes at, 14, 52–54, 115, 185, 186–87; compliance demonstrated by, 188; Comprehensive Risk Counseling Services at, 61–62, 150; confidentiality of, 48–49, 51, 62, 88–89; disconnecting of clients from, 185–86; events of, 120–24, 133; food pantry of, 64, 65, 139; funding of, 54–55, 60, 138–39, 208n3; inability of, to meet need, 159–60; location of, 47–48; medical case management by, 58; nonmedical case management at, 62–64; non–Ryan White–funded programs of, 64–66; nutritional programs at, 64, 206n3; "one-stop-shopping" care at, 50; pastoral care program at, 64, 65–66; as payer of last resort, 51; pedagogical exercises of, 124–27; programs of, 54–66, 122–23; security of, 49; as social location, 12, 185; spending freezes at, 56, 139, 140; study supported by, 10–11; substance abuse program at, 59–61; survival of, 118, 124–25; volunteerism at, 140–42, 144, 151–53, 161

Health Resources and Services Administration (HRSA), 118

highly active antiretroviral therapy (HAART), 31, 163

Hill, Benjamin, 19

HIV/AIDS: activism, 27–28; betrayal of citizens with, 24; comparison of, to other diseases, 166, 172; as "deserved," 27; diagnosis of, 84, 97, 104, 168, 170–71; as disease of the "other," 27, 28; empowerment of clients with, 22; as "equal-opportunity" disease, 28–30; "living well with," 33, 34; as medical event, 21, 44, 164–65; mortality of, 24, 30, 31, 34; in nonmembers of "risk groups," 27; in popular culture, 33–34, 40; rates of, among African Americans, 34–35, 39–40; research of, 28, 30–33, 208n2; risk counseling programs for, 61–62, 150, 201; as a social problem, 54; in South, 39–40, 41–42; stigma of, 9, 26–27, 48–49, 88–89, 175–79, 209n4; and survival, 31, 32–33; symptoms of, 172–73, 180–81; testing for, 34; transmission of, 18, 61–62, 201; in undeveloped and developed countries, 165; in women, 28; in women of color, 27

homelessness, 79; and social devaluation, 157–58; social networks and, 87–88, 154, 176; technical, 85

home ownership, 108, 185

homophobia, 27

Horton, Sarah, 116

housing: abuse and, 87–88; criminal record and, 82; eligibility for, 71, 82; indebtedness and, 100–102; loss of possessions and, 93–94, 102–3, 147, 176; and moves, 92–96, 100–101, 102–3, 176; poor conditions of, 91, 94, 147; rental payments for, as percentage of income, 78, 103; stability and, 78; vandalism and, 111. *See also* rooming and boardinghouses

Housing and Urban Development (HUD), 90

surveillance, 44

survival, 188–90; as behavioral improvement, 44, 123–24, 130–62; biomedical perspectives of, 163–83; daily life and, 15; definitions of, 6, 17–19; deservedness and, 25, 123, 127; discourse of, 22; as disempowering, 189–90; ethnography of, 3, 17–22; policies for, 22, 23–45; as public health goal, 31; as "socially productive," 25, 189; stories of, 19

survival strategies, 6, 18

Susser, Ida, 205n1

Tamara, 166–67, 168–69, 185

Tanya, 90–92, 173, 186

Tasha, 86–87, 157, 177, 178–79

taxes, assistance based on, 96

Taylor, 56

Temporary Assistance to Needy Families, 38, 90–91, 202, 203

thankfulness, 129, 130, 134, 135–37

therapeutic citizens, 5, 170

transportation assistance, 67

travel, affording, 143–44

Treatment Extension Act of 2009, 188

Treatment Modernization Act of 2006 (TMA), 2, 39–44, 47, 130–31, 203–4; clients' distrust of, 57; educational programs of, 117–28; fiscal oversight as aim of, 124, 126–27, 203; medical case management and, 58, 163–83; neoliberal rhetoric of, 43–44, 146, 148, 188; reimbursement procedures for, 55, 138–39, 207n8, 208n3. *See also* Ryan White CARE Act

Treichler, Paula, 25

Treva, 75, 96–98, 172, 186

tuition assistance, 69–70

Twelve Step Programs, 209n1

unemployment, 4, 37

U.S. Department of Health and Human Services (USDHHS), 2, 26

Veiled Sentiments (Abu-Lughod), 15

violence: disclosure of HIV status and, 176–77; experience of, by care providers, 52; experience of, by clients, 12, 86, 174, 176–77

viral load test, 206n1

vocational rehabilitation (VR), 69–70, 108, 204

volunteerism: benefits of, 142; degrading aspects of, 153; precariously situated women and, 151–53; responsibility proved by, 140–43, 153; skills for, 140–42; strategic, 109; vulnerable women shut out of, 161

vulnerable women, 80–89; blood work and, 179–81; definition of, 79; and disclosure of HIV status, 175–79; and empathy, 154–55; ineligibility of, for services, 154, 181; Medicaid and, 156–59; medical perspectives of, 175–81; social networks of, 86–87, 175; social network surrogacy of, 154–62

War on Poverty, 35

welfare: and biosocial inclusion, 165; eligibility limits on, 40, 51; and mandate to work, 38–39; moving off of, 38–39; racism and, 36; reform of, 4, 20, 35–39, 202;

Ronald Reagan on, 36; and
women of color, 36, 38
"welfare queen," 36, 38
*What Crazy Looks Like on an Ordinary
Day* (Cleage), 33
"White metaphor," 15
Women, Infants, and Children (WIC),
204

women with HIV/AIDS. *See* clients
work: as added stress, 92; difficulty
finding and keeping, 67–68;
strenuousness of, 83; and
vocational rehabilitation, 69–70;
welfare reform and, 4, 38–39, 202

Zivoudine. *See* azidothymidine (AZT)

In the Anthropology of Contemporary North America series:

Holding On: African American Women Surviving HIV/AIDS
Alyson O'Daniel

To order or obtain more information on these or other
University of Nebraska Press titles, visit nebraskapress.unl.edu.

CPSIA information can be obtained
at www.ICGtesting.com
Printed in the USA
LVOW07s1702081117
555515LV00003B/233/P